COMMON DISEASES

5th Edition

COMMON DISEASES

Their Nature, Prevalence and Care

5th Edition

by

John Fry
General Practitioner
Beckenham, Kent

and

Gerald Sandler
Consultant Physician Emeritus
Trent Regional Health Authority

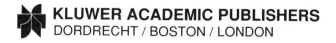
KLUWER ACADEMIC PUBLISHERS
DORDRECHT / BOSTON / LONDON

Distributors

for the United States and Canada: Kluwer Academic Publishers, PO Box 358, Accord Station, Hingham, MA 02018-0358, USA
for all other countries: Kluwer Academic Publishers Group, Distribution Center, PO Box 322, 3300 AH Dordrecht, The Netherlands

A catalogue record for this book is available from the British Library

ISBN 0-7923-8803-8

Library of Congress Cataloging-in-Publication Data

Fry, John, 1922–
    Common diseases : their nature, prevalence, and care / by John Fry
and Gerald Sandler. — 5th ed.
        p.   cm.
    Includes bibliographical references and index.
    ISBN 0-7923-8803-8 (casebound)
    1. Family medicine. 2. Diseases. I. Sandler, Gerald, 1928–
II. Title.
    [DNLM: 1. Disease. 2. Medicine. WB 100 F946c 1993]
    RC46.F94 1993
    616—dc20
    DNLM/DLC
    for Library of Congress   93-12605
                                                                          CIP

Copyright

Published in the United Kingdom by Kluwer Academic Publishers, PO Box 55, Lancaster, UK.

Kluwer Academic Publishers BV incorporates the publishing programmes of D. Reidel, Martinus Nijhoff, Dr. W. Junk and MTP Press.

Typeset by Keygraphics, Aldermaston, Berks.
Printed and bound in Great Britain by Hartnolls Ltd, Bodmin, Cornwall

CONTENTS

PREFACE

Common diseases commonly occur,
Rare diseases rarely happen!

In fact common diseases occur everywhere and in all fields of medicine but their 'commonness' varies with the field of practice.

It is particularly in primary care, family medicine or general practice that the true common diseases are really seen and managed, and it is to the general specialist levels at the district general hospitals that common problems are referred.

Familiarity has bred contempt towards common diseases – they are neglected by teachers, under-researched, little understood and managed with uncertainty and often with considerable lack of common sense.

What is new in this edition? For this fifth edition we aim to present our views on the common diseases as seen in primary and secondary medical care. The first four editions were based on the personal data of one GP over many years. Now in this fifth edition there is a new approach, a combination of a generalist primary physician and a general specialist.

We have selected the more important common diseases and for each one we follow a holistic sequence bringing together our joint clinical experiences together with epidemiology and outcomes. Thus for each condition we include

- What is it?
- Who gets it and when?
- How does it present?
- What happens and with what outcomes?
- What to do?

The clinical sections have been considerably expanded, as we firmly believe that many of the common medical problems encountered in primary care can be diagnosed and managed on the basis of a good clinical history and examination. We have added new simple line drawings where we consider them helpful in defining and clarifying clinical features in the various conditions. Regrettably, the current increasing pressure for 'high technology' medicine may well lead to an inadequate emphasis on the value and importance of the basic clinical skills in deciding diagnosis and management, and it is our hope that this book may help in some small measure to redress this balance.

We have also tried to update current views on aetiology where appropriate, as well as highlighting new approaches in investigation and treatment of the various conditions described. So, for example, we have discussed new views on the role of *Helicobacter pyloridis* in the aetiology of peptic ulcer, the importance of free oxygen radicals in ageing, the multifactorial origin of rheumatoid arthritis, new views on the aetiology of migraine, diabetes and viral hepatitis, chemical markers in the early diagnosis of cancer of the gastrointestinal tract, when to consider surgery in patients with angina and how to investigate them, the place of fibrinolysis in the management of myocardial infarction, especially in the context of primary care, the 'block' treatment of thyrotoxicosis, and the use of sumatriptan in migraine. In describing these medical advances since the fourth edition of this book, we have also tried to put them in perspective in relation to primary care, and we hope that this approach will be useful.

We dedicate this new book to all those who manage common diseases! In particular, to general practitioners and family physicians and the primary care team, but also to general specialists and, of course, to teachers and students.

Common diseases are not parochial and they have no national boundaries. They are similar in all countries. Sitting in on colleagues in Europe, North America and the Far East one of us (J.F.) found the same common conditions and therefore we include them in our dedication.

Although between us we have almost 100 years of clinical experience nevertheless we acknowledge our limits and hope that this book will stimulate others to study common diseases more extensively.

John Fry
Gerald Sandler

SECTION I

COMMON DISEASES

CLINICAL DISEASES

CHAPTER **1**

HEALTH, DISEASE, CARE

'To cure sometimes, to relieve often, to comfort always and to prevent hopefully'

It is well to begin with a sense of realistic humility and to remind ourselves that even in our present state of advanced medical technology:

- we can *cure* only *sometimes* and that in general practice dramatic specific cures are infrequent;
- certainly our potentials for *relief* are great with wide scope for medication and physical methods;
- as caring physicians with access and availability for patients to consult us, we must endeavour to use each consultation as an opportunity for *support and comfort*;
- whilst *prevention* of disease must be a goal, it must be realized that the physician's roles must be to motivate and educate patients about their own responsibilities for health maintenance as well as organizing primary prevention programmes.

What is 'health'?

Health as defined by the World Health Organization – 'a state of complete physical, mental and social wellbeing and not merely an

3

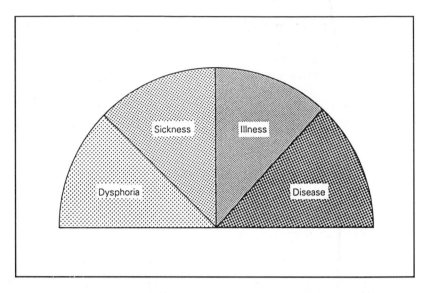

Fig. 1.1—Spectrum of 'non-health'

absence of disease' – is a rare, personal and subjective state experienced by less than 1 in 10 of the population at any time; nevertheless, it has to be a Utopian goal.

What is 'non-health'?

The converse of health is *non-health* with a wide spectrum of grades of severity.

It ranges from a feeling of *dysphoria* or general dissatisfaction with one's life; through *sickness* when the person feels that there is something wrong requiring some relief by self-care measures (note that on any day one-third of the population takes some over-the-counter medicines); *illness* which is a state requiring advice from a health professional, usually a GP consultation in the UK; to a *disease* or a diagnostic label applied by a physician, and diseases can be graded into minor, chronic and major (see pages 26–29).

Whose responsibilities?

Responsibilities for health maintenance and promotion, disease prevention and management must be shared between *individuals* and *families* who must accept and adopt the rules for good health, such as avoiding health risks (e.g. smoking), regular exercise, sensible diet, drinking in moderation and collaborating in organized disease prevention programmes; *professionals* – doctors and nurses – who, in addition, to traditional disease management, should use the opportunities of a consultation for health education; and the *providers*, the National Health Service in the UK or government and insurance organizations in other countries. All involved have to pay attention to ensuring optimal economic efficiency and effectiveness.

What factors?

Underlying the causation, nature, progression and outcome of disease are a multiplicity of factors:

- *clinical* – specific causes and pathologies and response to treatment;
- *social* – income, housing, lifestyles, occupation, literacy, safe water, food and environment;
- *personal* – such as family and genetic traits and susceptibilities. It is well known in practice that apart from known genetic inherited liabilities certain families are more prone to suffer from particular conditions and with higher consultation rates, demands and expectations.

What is disease?

As noted, a disease is a diagnostic objective label attached by a professional, such as a physician or nurse. It is arrived at following a recognized process of symptom assessment, examination and investigation.

There are international classifications of disease which attempt to cover the whole range of possible specific diseases and symptoms. However, in the real-life clinical situations of general practice an accurate and confirmed specific diagnosis is often impossible, and it must be accepted that a general knowledge and experience of symptoms and syndromes and, more particularly, of individual family characteristics gathered over years, often are more important than disease-labelling.

What are the common diseases?

'Common diseases commonly occur,
rare diseases rarely happen'

The 'commonness' of disease depends on the field and place of work. Thus, the common diseases seen by a neurologist are different from those of a general physician (internist), which will be different from those of primary care.

Three factors influence the nature and prevalence of common diseases:

(1) *The size of the population* (i.e. the denominator). Thus, the likely frequency of disease in a general practice population of 2000 per GP principal will be very different from that seen by his specialist colleagues at a local district general hospital responsible for over ¼ million. For example, a GP can expect 3–4 cases of acute appendicitis in a year, whereas the local general surgical teams will deal with 300–400. A GP can expect only one new cancer of the lung and one new cancer of the breast each year, whereas the local hospitals will see over 100 of each type annually. However, the general practitioner will see hundreds of patients with respiratory infections, high blood pressure, emotional problems and aches and pains, few of which are seen by specialists (see page 20).

(2) *Pre-selection.* In the British NHS the referral system ensures a filtering mechanism between primary and secondary care. There is no direct access to specialists as in some other health systems. Thus, the general practitioner refers only those patients which require specialist care and therefore most of the common diseases in the community will not be seen by specialists.

(3) *Time changes.* No disease is static. Over time there occur changes in prevalence and severity. Thus, rheumatic fever is very uncommon now, whereas 40–50 years ago each GP saw a few cases each year. Tuberculosis is rare; in the 1950s I (J.F.) had 3–4 patients with tuberculosis under my care at any time. Now I have not seen a patient with TB for over 15 years. Poliomyelitis has disappeared as has smallpox; cancer of the lung has become more frequent, there are more older persons with degenerative disorders, and asthma is being diagnosed more frequently.

The severity of some diseases has changed; otitis media, although as frequent, now has few serious complications and peptic ulcers are less frequent and less troublesome. The reasons for changes are multiple, such as more effective treatments, but also changes in the causes and the hosts.

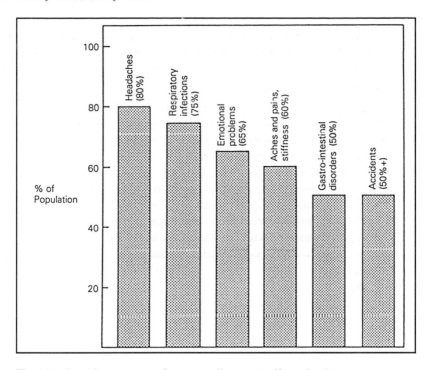

Fig. 1.2—Annual occurrence of common diseases at self-care level

Common diseases

At the basic *family level of self-care*, there are few persons who have a year free from disease or symptoms. Thus, in a year:

- 80% have headaches;
- 75% of adults suffer from one or more respiratory infections (common cold, sore throat, chest infection);
- 65% admit to suffering from depression, anxiety, headaches, tiredness and other emotional problems;
- 60% have various aches, pains, backache, joint stiffness or arthritis;
- 50% suffer from various gastro-intestinal disorders;
- more than one-half sustain some accident.

In *general practice*, the common diseases are shown by the proportions of persons in a practice who will consult their GP in a year:

- 27% will consult for a respiratory infection;
- 16% for various 'symptoms' without a specific diagnosis;
- 10% for disorders of the nervous system, ears or eyes;
- 10% for musculo-skeletal disorders;
- 10% for non-respiratory infections;
- 10% for minor accidents;
- 10% for psycho-emotional problems;
- 7% for cardiovascular diseases;
- 10% for preventive and health promotional activities.

Note: persons may consult for more than 1 category)

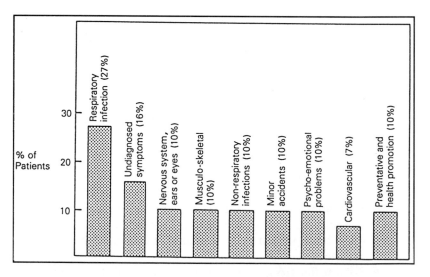

Fig. 1.3—common diseases as shown by proportions of persons in a practice who consult their GP in a year

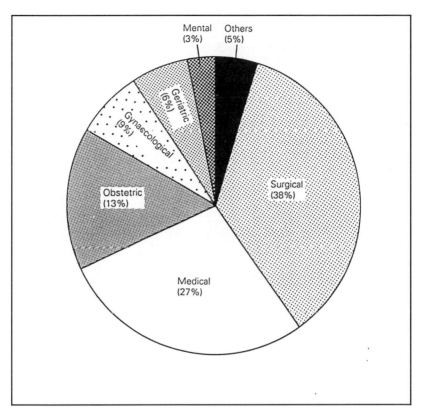

Fig. 1.4—Distribution of admissions to a district general hospital

At a *district general hospital* the distribution of admissions will be:

- surgical   38%
  general   15%
  trauma and orthopaedic   9%
  ear, nose, throat   4%
  urology   3%
  ophthalmology   2%
  other   5%
- medical   25%
  general   14%
  paediatric   7%
  other   4%
- obstetric   13%
- gynaecology   9%
- geriatric   6%
- mental   3%
- others   5%

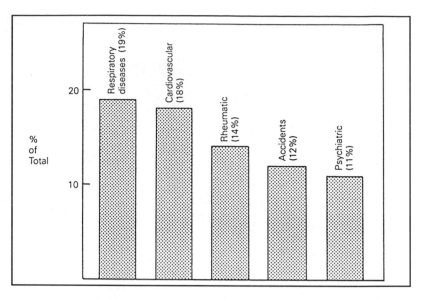

Fig. 1.5—Most frequent causes of certified spells of absence from work

The most frequent causes of *certified spells of sickness – absence from work*:

- respiratory diseases   19%
- cardiovascular   18%
- rheumatic   14%
- accidents   12%
- psychiatric   11%

The *common causes of death*:

- circulatory system   54%
  ischaemic heart disease   31%
  strokes   14%
- neoplasms   28%
- respiratory system   12%

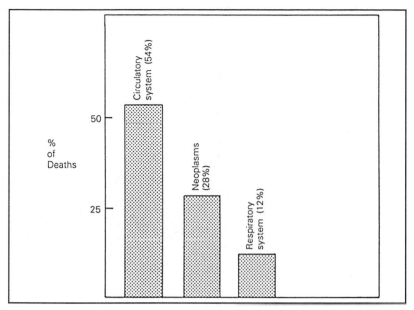

Fig. 1.6—The common causes of death

Basic questions

For a proper understanding of disease in man and man in disease five questions should be asked and answered for each disease:

What is it?

It is axiomatic that we should know the nature, causes and pathology of the disease, but this may be uncertain for many major as well as minor conditions. We are uncertain of causes and nature of high blood pressure and arthritis as well as the common cold and depression. Nevertheless, the physician has to create his own understanding in order to proceed.

Who gets it and when?

Most diseases have characteristic patterns of age and sex incidence and prevalence. Thus, some occur in children, some in young adults, some in mid-age and many more in old age.

What happens?

A knowledge of the likely course and outcome of a disease is important. This has to be more than a 'prognosis'. It must be an appreciation of the *natural history of the disease*. There are five patterns (Figure 1.7):

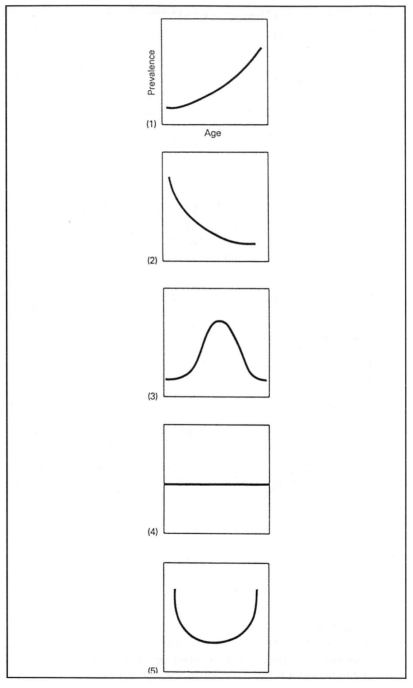

Fig. 1.7—Disease patterns: (1) ageing, (2) childhood, (3) adult, (4) persistent, (5) diseases of young and old

(1) Diseases that are associated with the *ageing process*, becoming more frequent and more serious with age – as cancer, heart disease, strokes.

(2) Diseases of *childhood* – many disappear as the child grows up, i.e. common respiratory infections, asthma, otitis media and certain orthopaedic and skin disorders.

(3) Diseases of *young adults and middle age* which 'come and go'; that is they appear, cause considerable problems and then apparently subside. In this group are migraine, acute backs, duodenal ulcer, irritable bowel syndrome, asthma, hay fever, acute urinary tract infections in women, and anxiety–depression (to some extent).

(4) Some *congenital* and other diseases once present remain unchanged throughout life.

(5) A small number of conditions are most prevalent in *young and old*, such as herniae, hydrocoele and constipation.

How does it present?

Clinical experience teaches that a specific disease may present in different guises which have to be noted and elucidated.

What to do?

This is the ultimate decision facing the physician. Having made a probable diagnosis there are another set of questions: Are further investigations necessary? Can I deal with it or does the patient need referral? Is treatment urgent or can the decision be delayed? What specific treatment should be given and for what purposes? When should the patient be seen again to check on progress and outcome?

Care

Systems of care

Health care is a human right and all countries provide some. There is no single 'best-buy' system that can be applied to all countries because each develops in relation to national characteristics, such as political, historical and economic philosophies, wealth, religion, geography, literacy, education and social conditions.

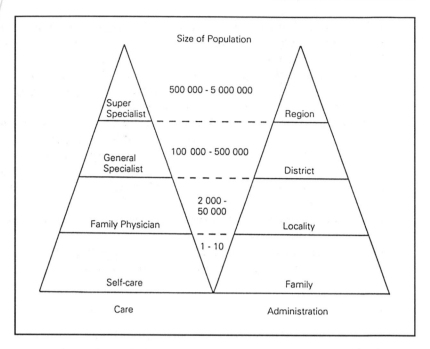

Fig. 1.8—Levels of care

Thus, the *US* has a health system based on free enterprise and personal insurance; *Western European countries* rely on a mixture of government and compulsory social and health insurance; *UK and Scandinavian countries* have more comprehensive systems financed largely out of general taxation; and the *socialist countries* set up national bureaucratic systems run by central and local governments.

Structure

Within every system there are four essential recognizable levels of care, each with its own roles and functions and needs for skills, resources, training and information. Also, each relate to *care, population size* and *administration* (Figure 1.8).

Levels

- *Self-care* where persons manage their own health problems in the context of a *family*, which in the UK now averages 4, 2 parents and 2 children.

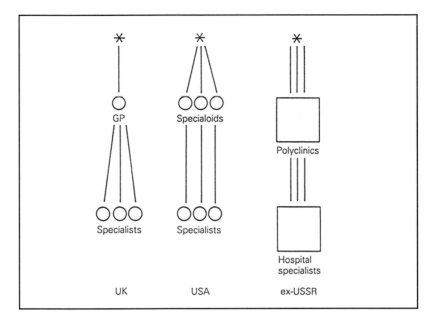

Fig. 1.9—Flow of care

- *Primary professional care* provides the first contact once a person decides that professional advice is needed. In the UK this is a *general practitioner* (GP), with whom the person/family are registered, but in other systems it may be a specialoid, the local hospital or a specialist to whom there is free access and choice. The GP cares for about *2000* patients and works in a *local neighbourhood.*
- *General specialist care* is based at local *district* general hospitals, each serving a population of about *250 000* people. In the UK patients are selectively referred to such hospitals with general specialities such as surgery, medicine, paediatrics, trauma and orthopaedics, OBG, psychiatry and others.
- *Super (sub) specialist care,* such as neurology, neurosurgery, cardio-thoracic surgery, renal dialysis and transplants and others, is based at *regional* units serving 1–5 million people. Cases are referred to them most usually from the districts, but sometimes direct from general practice.

Thus, each level has a different population size and as noted (pages 6–10) the *common* disease problems will be very different.

Flow of care

Another way of looking at a health system is to note what happens when a person or family seek medical care – where and to whom do they go?

In the *UK* there is a single portal of entry into the NHS through the *GP* who decides when referral to specialists is necessary.

In the *USA* the family has to select a *'specialoid'* for consultation, such as an internist, paediatrician, OBG, psychiatrist, etc. who may combine primary and secondary care or refer to a *specialist*.

In the *USSR* (that was) there is no free choice – persons are allocated to a *neighbourhood uchastok doctor* in a polyclinic who provides primary care, or they may go direct to a *polyclinic specialoid* who may refer to a *hospital specialist*.

Extent of care

- Most care is *self-care*.
- Out of all symptoms, 75% are managed by the family.
- Only 1 problem in 4 is taken to a *GP* in the UK, and the GP will seek a referral to a hospital specialist in only 5–10% of all consultations (Figure 1.10) (see also page 20).

What is general practice?

General practice in the NHS has roles and features that are distinct from hospital practice.

- GP provides *direct access and availability* to registered patients, who may be selectively referred to hospitals.
- GP provides *first-contact care* which demands analysis and assessment of packages of undefined symptoms presented by patients; those referred to hospitals are pre-packaged with a diagnosis and referred to a special department.
- GP provides care for a relatively *small (2000 average) and stable population*; a district general hospital (DGH) serves 250 000, which means 125 GPs relating to a DGH which may have 50–100 various hospital specialists.
- GP provides *long-term and continuing care* possibly over many years; DGH provides episodic care to transient patients.
- The *morbidity spectrum* of a general practice will be that of 2000 persons per GP: that of a DGH will be selected from 250 000.

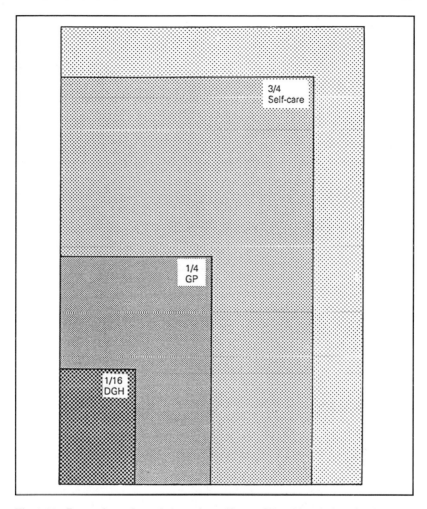

Fig. 1.10—Proportions of population using self-care, GP and hospital services in a year

The GP serves as a personal and *family adviser, philosopher and friend* to patients over many years; as a *gatekeeper* to the hospital; a *protector* of the hospital against unnecessary cases and protector of patients against unnecessary hospital care; and as a *coordinator* and *manipulator* of community services for his/her patients.

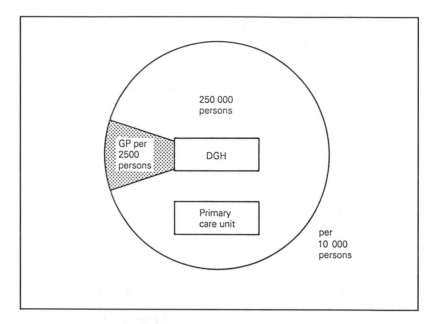

Fig. 1.11—District care

Some national demographic facts

- Population of UK = 57.7 million
  under 15 = 19%
  over 65 = 16%
- Birth rate = 13.4 per 1000 (*note*: 25% to unmarried mothers)
- Infant mortality = 8.6 per 1000 births
- Death rate = 11.9 per 1000
- Fertility rate = 1.8 (average number of children per woman of 15–45)
- Life expectancies (at birth) = Male 73 years
  Female 79 years

What does this data mean? Our population is almost stable now with less than 2 children per couple. The proportion of over 65s has been rising and will continue to do so as our life expectancies go up.

- *Household size* has been decreasing and averages 2.6 persons, with one-quarter single persons, one-third 2 person households and one-third 3 and 4 person households.

- *Carers*: 1 in 8 adults are providing care for a disabled dependent.
- *Marriages* are 6.7 per 1000.
- *Divorces* are 2.9 per 1000 – suggesting that 1 in 3 of marriages may end in divorce.
- 14 per cent of *children* live in single-parent households.

Social features

- *Smoking* is decreasing faster in men than women:
  Men – 35% smoke;
  Women – 31% smoke.
  There are wide differences in social classes:
  social class I – 18% smoke;
  social class V – 40% smoke.
- *Alcohol* (average) consumption per week:
  Men – 15 units (25 units in 18–25 age);
  Women – 5 units.
  (*Note*: 15% men and 2% women consume more than 35 units per week.)

NHS data

- *Costs*
  In 1991–2 the cost of the NHS will be *£35 billion*. This means *£600 per head* of the population.
  In terms of *GNP* the NHS cost is 5.85% and the cost of private care and self-medication a further 1.02%. Total UK health cost is 6.9% GNP.
- *Funding – sources*
  85% from general taxation
  10% from National Health Insurance contributions
  5% from direct charges for prescriptions, etc.
- *Where does money go?*
  hospitals   60%
  general medical services   20% (GPs 8% and prescribing 12%)
  other   20%
- *NHS manpower*
  More than 1 million persons are employed in NHS
  nurses   500 000
  doctors   90 000
- *Doctors* (1992 estimates)
  Hospital
     consultants   20 000
     junior hospital doctors   35 000

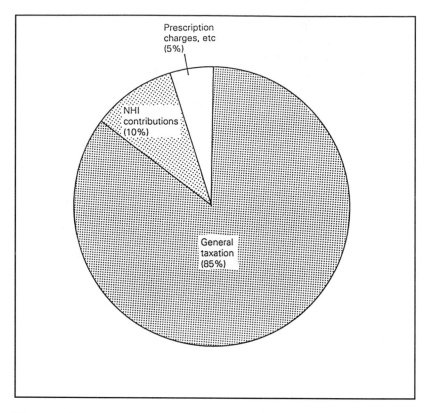

Fig. 1.12—Sources of NHS funding

GPs
  principals   33 000
  assistants   300
  trainees   1 900
• *Hospital beds*   5.5 per 1000 population
• *Hospital annual utilization of population*
inpatients (deaths and discharges) 13%
new outpatient referrals   18%
A-E attendances   23%
These rates for hospital utilization may include some persons
in more than one of the three categories, but they do suggest
that about 1 in 3 of the population uses NHS hospitals in any
year.

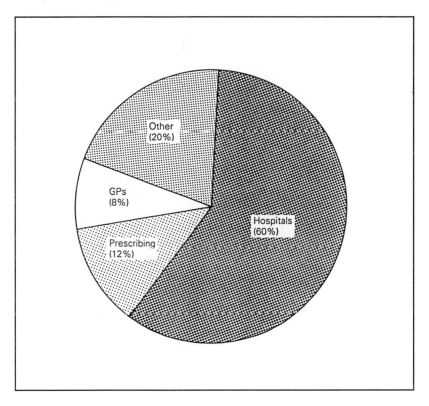

Fig. 1.13—Where NHS money goes

- *General practice*
  The number of *NHS GP principals* has increased by 1.5% a year over the past 20 years, which means by about 450 per year.
  As a consequence with a fairly static population, the average *list size* per GP has fallen from 2500 in the 1960s to 1875 in 1992 (1500 in Scotland).

Practices

A major change in the past 25 years has been the trend towards larger partnerships and units.

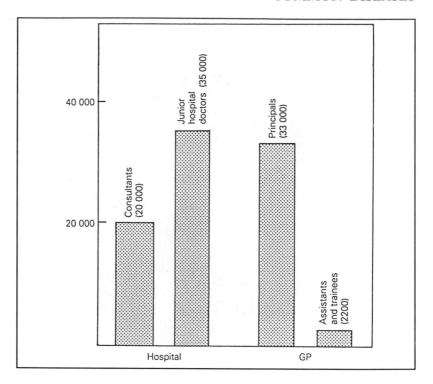

Fig. 1.14—Doctors employed by NHS (1992 estimates)

single handed	10%
2 partners	12%
3 partners	17%
4 partners	19%
5 partners	18%
6 partners and over	24%

Practice team

Along with larger practice groups has come the buildup of the practice team and a typical model might consists of –

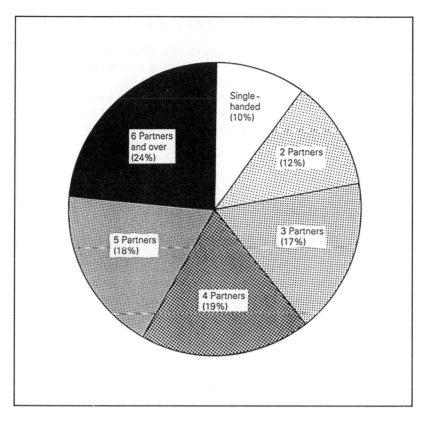

Fig. 1.15—Practice sizes – distribution of all GPs

GPs	5
Manager	1
Receptionists	10
Secretaries and computer operators	4
Practice nurses	4
Attached	
District nurses	3
Health visitors	2
Community midwives	2
Social workers	2
Total	33

What goes on in a practice? A bird's eye view

A *practice profile* of numbers, events, work, content and actions is a useful exercise, not only for learning and teaching, but also as a means of audit and annual report.

Since most GPs now work in groups, the presentation should include likely experience of an individual GP with 2000 patients and a group with 10 000.

Practice populations

TABLE 1.1 Approximate age distributions of patients in single and group practices

Age	under 5	5–14	15–29	30–44	45–64	65–74	75–84	85+	Total
Per GP	140	240	440	420	440	180	110	30	2 000
Per group	700	1200	2200	2100	2200	900	550	150	10 000

Demography

TABLE 1.2 Annual births, deaths and associated events

	Per GP (2000)	Per group (10 000)
Births		
Outcome of pregnancy		
natural	22	110
assisted	3	15
Caesarean section	3	15
Total	28	140
Abortions		
terminations of pregnancy	5	25
spontaneous abortions	5	25
Total	10	50
Deaths		
in hospital	16	80
at home	5	25
in hospice	1	5
elsewhere	1	5
Total	23	115

Work patterns

It is possible to construct theoretical estimates of likely volume and time of work.

Volume of work

70% of persons will consult their GP in a year: that is, 1400 out of the average list size of 2000 (patient consulting rate) or 7000 in a 10 000 person practice

Although the average *annual consultation rate per person* varies with practices and with GPs, the average rates are between 3 and 4 consultations (i.e. total consultations and home visits divided by population).

Thus, it is possible to produce likely work rates from a practice population of 2000 with these two rates (Table 1.3). Home visits now represent 10% of contacts.

TABLE 1.3 Likely GP work rates

	Practice population 2000	
	Annual consultation rate of 3	Annual consultation rate of 4
Per year		
Office consultations	5400	7200
Home visits	600	800
Total	6000	8000
Per week		
Office consultations	104	138
Home visits	12	15
Total	116	153
Per day (5 day week)		
Office consultations	21	27
Home visits	2	3
Total	23	30

Table 1.3 suggests that the *basic* daily volume of consultations and home visits will be between 23 and 30 contacts. In addition, there are other duties and tasks for GPs, such as administration, telephone, correspondence, writing prescriptions, learning and teaching and consulting with partners and specialists.

At present there are 38 claims for *night visits* (10 pm – 8am) per GP annually, that is less than 1 per week.

The Doctors and Dentists Pay Review Body in collaboration with the General Medical Services of BMA reported on *average work and time per week* for GPs. They found:

General medical duties	37.01 hours
Other tasks	4.97 hours
On call	23.48 hours
Total	65.46 hours

Thus, for those GPs who are on an on-call rota the week will be over 65 hours: if on-call time is excluded, the total is almost 42 hours; and for general medical services it is 37 hours.

Face-to-face consultations and home visits (including travel time) will amount to around 27 hours per week.

Morbidity content

What can the GP in an average practice expect to see in a year? One way of presenting the facts is to show how many patients in a practice of 2000 and a group of 10 000 are likely to consult in a year for various disorders. (The data is composite from J.F.'s own practice and the *Third National Study of Morbidity Statistics from General Practice 1981–2*, published HMSO 1986, and from HMSO Social Trends publications 1980–1991). The grades of disease problems that present in practice are:

Specific minor	52%
Chronic (intermediate)	33%
Major	15%

(*Note*: Social issues involve 1 in 3 of consultations).

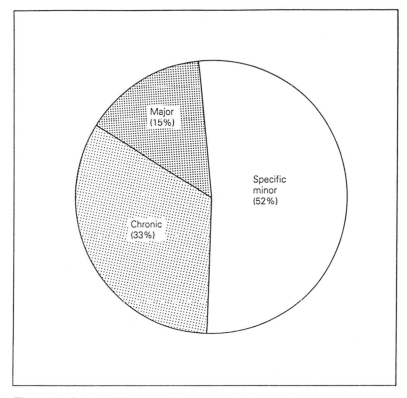

Fig. 1.16—Grades of disease problems presenting in practice

The most common disease groups (%) of all patients who consult in a year:

- Respiratory infections   30%
- Skin disorders   15%
- Musculo-skeletal   12%
- Psychiatric   10%
- Gastro-intestinal   7%

It should be noted, however, that in addition 20% of patients will attend for preventive and health promotional activities, such as immunization, cervical smears, family planning, antenatal care, travel advice, general checkup and examinations and certification.

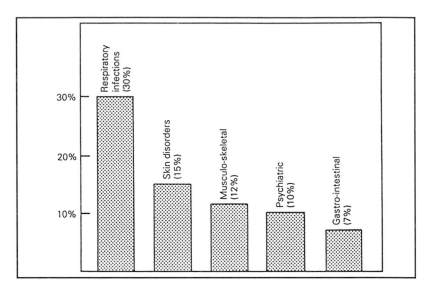

Fig. 1.17—The most common disease groups in general practice

The numbers in the various grades and categories are given in the following tables.

TABLE 1.4   Specific minor conditions – numbers consulting

Condition	Annual persons consulting	
	per 2000	per 10 000
Psycho-emotional	150	750
Acute throat infections	120	600
Backache	120	600
Eczema–dermatitis	100	500
Acute otitis media	92	460
Otitis externa	22	110
Ear wax	46	230
Urinary tract infections (male and female)	60	300
Dyspepsia	44	225
Migraine/headache	50	250
Hay fever	40	200
Vertigo/dizzy	30	150
Varicose veins	27	135
Constipation	18	90
Piles	16	80
Hernia	16	80

(*Note*: there may be more than one condition per person)

TABLE 1.5 Chronic conditions – numbers consulting

Condition	Annual persons consulting	
	per 2000	per 10 000
Cardiovascular		
High blood pressure	100	500
Chronic heart failure	24	120
(various causes)		
Anaemia	20	100
(pernicious anaemia)	(3)	(12)
Central nervous system		
Strokes (effects)	20	100
Epilepsy	12	60
Parkinsonism	4	20
Multiple sclerosis	2	10
Cancers		
New	8	40
(under care)	(15)	(75)
Respiratory		
Asthma	40	200
Chronic bronchitis /		
emphysema	50	250
Gastro-intestinal		
Peptic ulcers	12	60
Irritable bowel syndrome	24	120
Diverticular disease	4	20
Endocrine		
Diabetes	20	100
Thyroid	11	55
Chronic renal failure	1	4
Psychiatric (chronic)	50	250

TABLE 1.6 Major diseases – numbers consulting

Condition	Annual persons consulting	
	per 2000	per 10 000
Acute chest infections		
Acute bronchitis	116	580
Pneumonia	12	60
Acute myocardian infarction	8	40
(sudden death)	(4)	(20)
Acute strokes	6	30
Severe depression	10	50
(Suicide)	(1 in 6 years)	(1)
Acute abdomen	6	30
New cancers	8	40

Social pathology

In addition to medical diseases, there is much social pathology in the community.

TABLE 1.7   Social pathology

Situation	Persons affected in year	
	per 2000	per 10 000
Poverty (grants)	300	1500
Unemployed	90	450
Homeless ('official')	5	25
One parent families	30	150
Marriages	13	65
Divorces	5	25
Terminations of pregnancy	5	25
Crime		
In prison	2	10
Burglaries	35	175
Drunken drivers	5	25
Sexual assault	1	5

Disabilities

Recording only numbers of patients who consult omits appreciation of the many who are disabled and who do *not* consult. Table 1.8 gives approximate numbers in population of 2000 and 10 000 from community surveys supported by the Royal College of Physicians. There are two grades – those who have any disability and those who are severely disabled.

TABLE 1.8   Disabilities

Disability	per 2000		per 10 000	
	Total	Severe +	Total	Severe +
Rheumatic				
Osteoarthritis	580	} 10	2900	} 50
Rheumatoid arthritis	50		250	
Cardiac				
IHD	} 140	7	} 700	35
Heart failure				
Respiratory				
Respiratory	160	20	800	100
CNS				
Stroke (survivors)	11	3	55	15
Severe head injury	3	3	15	15
Parkinsonism	4	1	20	5
Multiple sclerosis	2	1	8	4
Motor neurone disease	< 1	—	1	1
Muscular dystrophy	< 1	—	1	1
Epilepsy	10	1	50	5
Continence				
Regular urinary				
incontinence	88	8	440	40
Colostomy	3	—	15	1
Amputations				
(lower limb)	2	—	11	—
(upper limb)	< 1	—	2	—
Congenital				
Congenital (at birth)	40	4	200	20

From RCP (1986) *Physical Disability in 1986 and Beyond* and own practice

Practical points

- Each system of health care has four levels each with its own roles, tools, skills and needs for education and training, and its own set of 'common diseases'.
- For effective management of any disease, it is necessary to know:
  What is it?
  Who gets it when?
  How does it present?
  What happens?
  What to do and why and with what outcome?
- In the UK there is a fairly static population with low fertility rate and birth rate, an ageing population, with high divorce rates and 25% of births to unmarried mothers.
- The annual cost of NHS is £600 per head and general practice accounts for 20%, including prescribing.
- Number of GPs has been increasing by almost 2% a year (over 500) and list sizes per GP have fallen (now 1875 per GP).
- About one-third of the population uses hospital services every year.
- Practice team size has been growing and a group practice of 5 GPs now includes over 30 members.
- There are 28 births per GP a year, almost all in hospital, with a 10% Caesarean rate and 10% assisted deliveries.
- 65% of deaths occur in hospital and 25% at home.
- A GP with 2000 patients is likely to have 25–30 face-to-face consultations per day, plus other duties.
- It is estimated that a GP works a 65-hour week (including 'on-call') with 27 hours in consultations.
- 52% of disease in general practice is minor, 33% chronic–intermediate, and 12% major–serious.
- One-third of all work is with respiratory infections, with skin disorders, musculo-skeletal problems, psychiatric and gastro-intestinal conditions next in order.
- Most prevalent chronic conditions are hypertension, asthma and chronic bronchitis, central nervous system diseases and depression.
- Major diseases are uncommon. 8 new cancers a year per GP, 6 acute abdomens, 6 strokes, 8 myocardial infarctions and over 100 acute chest infections.
- These questions and issues concerning all these facts for each practice to note and discuss.

SECTION II

RESPIRATORY DISEASES

CHAPTER 2

RESPIRATORY DISEASES – THE CLINICAL SPECTRUM

Respiratory diseases are the most prevalent of common diseases all over the world.

This is not surprising since the respiratory tract is the easiest portal of entry to outside pathogens, irritants and pollutants. Since we breathe once roughly every 2 or 3 seconds, the opportunities for entry into the respiratory tract are great.

Patient consulting rates

Personal data and those from the 3rd National Morbidity Study show that as many as one-half of all persons may consult once or more times a year for a respiratory disorder (Table 2.1). However, the true proportion is less because some will consult for more than one diagnosis.

Consultation rates

Many common respiratory conditions are relatively benign and do not require more than one consultation per episode. Therefore, annual consultation rates are proportionately lower.

Respiratory conditions account for almost one-quarter (22%) of all consultations.

TABLE 2.1 Annual patient consulting rates

Condition	per 2000	per 10 000
Upper respiratory infection (URI)		
Acute URI	290	1450
Flu-like illness	34	170
Acute throat infections	120	600
Glandular fever (IM)	3	15
Total	447	2235
Acute chest infections		
Bronchitis	116	580
Pneumonia	12	60
Total	128	640
Chronic chest conditions		
Chronic bronchitis – emphysema	50	250
Asthma	40	200
Total	90	450
Ears		
Acute otitis media	92	460
Otitis externa	22	110
Wax	46	230
Vertigo – dizziness	10	50
Total	170	850
Nose		
Catarrh	40	200
Chronic sinus	4	20
Nose bleeds	8	40
Total	52	260
Hay fever	40	200
Cancer of lung	2	10
Chest pains	24	120
Others	40	200

Sickness–invalidity benefits

Respiratory disorders are the largest group of conditions causing absence from work or prolonged invalidity accounting for 25% of all causes.

• acute upper respiratory infections	5
• 'flu-like illness'	5
• 'bronchitis'	9
• asthma	3
• others	3
Total	25%

Hospital in-patient data

11% of all admissions and discharges from NHS hospitals were for respiratory conditions (93 per 10 000 of population).

Causes of death

Approximately 20% of all deaths are certified as due to some respiratory disease (119 300 out of 600 000). The numbers, in round figures are listed in Table 2.2.

TABLE 2.2 Deaths caused by respiratory disease

Cause	Annual deaths	%
Cancer of lung	40 000	34
Pneumonia	30 000	25
Bronchitis – emphysema	11 000	9
Asthma	2 300	2
Cor pulmonale	24 000	20
Others	12 000	10
Total	119 300	100

As with other groups, the accuracy of death certification is questionable for labels such as 'disorders of the pulmonary circulation' or 'cor pulmonale'.

Practical points

- It is likely that in a year between one-third and one-half of all persons consult for a respiratory condition.
- Most prevalent are:

	% of total
acute upper respiratory infections	48%
acute chest infections	14%
chronic chest conditions	4%
ears	18%
nasal	10%

- One-quarter of all certified absence from work and invalidity is due to respiratory diseases.
- 11% of hospital admissions and 20% of deaths are from respiratory diseases.

CHAPTER 3

ACUTE UPPER RESPIRATORY INFECTIONS AND INFLUENZA

Probably the largest group of common diseases in the world, nevertheless, the upper respiratory infections are a confusing mass of uncertainty of nature, causes and management.

Everyone suffers one or more attacks every year; some individuals and families appear more susceptible than others. Fortunately, whilst causing much discomfort and malaise they cause few complications and are self-limiting. Management, therefore, should be aimed at relief and comfort rather than at pseudo-attempts at cures.

Classification is difficult because of uncertainty of causation and poor correlation between possible specific pathogens and clinical features. Discussion, therefore, has to be based on broad clinical presentations in the chapters that follow, i.e.

- acute upper respiratory infections and influenza;
- catarrhal children;

- acute otitis media;
- acute throat infections and glandular fever (infectious mononucleosis).

Common colds and coughs

What are they?

In spite of global research over many years, clarification of the cause is elusive and even when some have been identified this is of little assistance in management.

It is assumed that common coughs and colds are caused by *viruses* and many have been named:

- rhinoviruses – responsible for common colds;
- adenoviruses – various respiratory infections;
- coronaviruses – various respiratory infections;
- Coxsackie A and B – colds, sore throats and Bornholm disease;
- respiratory syncytial viruses – annual epidemics of coughs and colds in children and bronchiolitis and pneumonia in infants;
- para-influenza – croup, coughs and colds in children;
- epidemic influenza – caused by specific viruses.

Bacteria are not primary causes of common colds and coughs but may cause secondary infections by *Streptococcus pyogenes*, *haemophilus influenzae* and *pneumococci*. It is difficult at times to separate these common infections from hyper-reactive nasal symptoms in individuals with vasomotor rhinitis.

Who gets them and when?

Although coughs and colds are most prevalent in mid-winter they occur throughout the year. Following a low incidence rate in the summer months the rate begins to rise a few weeks after schoolchildren return from summer holidays and reaches a peak (in the UK) from December to April.

As noted in Chapter 2 the annual patient consulting rate is 15%. The age incidence (Figure 3.1) shows that the consulting rates are highest in young children (0–4 years) and then decrease to low levels in adults.

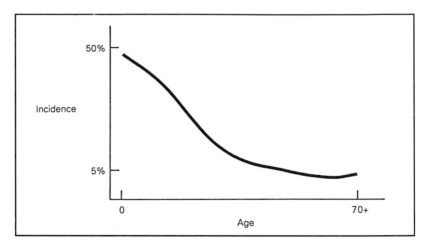

Fig. 3.1—Consulting rates for coughs and colds

How do they present?

The respiratory tract is a single contiguous unit from the nose to the lungs. The clinical presentation therefore may include variable degrees of:

- sneezing, nasal discharge and blockage;
- sore throat;
- cough;
- variable general malaise.

What happens?

The usual course is for natural resolution to occur within a week or two. An old clinical aphorism was that a common cold was '3 days coming, 3 days there and 3 days going'! However, it may be shorter or more prolonged.

Complications are unusual in normal healthy persons but certain individuals are more vulnerable such as chronic respiratory invalids with chronic bronchitis, fibrocystic disease, cardiac invalids, and persons with immune deficiency disorders.

What to do?

With such common conditions of uncertain causation and a benign self-limiting course the treatment protocol should be simple and safe avoiding pseudospecific potentially harmful drugs.

There are few indications for antibiotics and antihistamines.

Relief and comfort should be based on:

- simple explanation, advice and reassurance;
- simple analgesics;
- simple hot drinks, demulcent preparations, or inhalants.

Epidemic influenza and influenza-like illness

Distinction has to be made between epidemic influenza and influenza-like illness. *Real epidemics of influenza* occur infrequently every few years and are unmistakable clinically and nationally with large numbers of persons being affected and with many positive reports of isolations of specific influenza viruses.

Influenza-like illness or 'flu' is endemic and is a useful clinical label applied to common features, such as an upper respiratory infection accompanied by considerable malaise, aches and pains, and fever.

Epidemic influenza

What is it?

As noted, epidemics of influenza are caused by specific influenza viruses A, B or C. Influenza A viruses are responsible for the more extensive and virulent epidemics. They have the facility of continually changing strains by mutations in their haemagglutinin strains so that natural acquired immunity is difficult to maintain and vaccines offer only temporary protection and have to be changed continually.

World pandemics of influenza with new strains of exceptional virulence seem to have occurred about once every 10 years over the past three centuries. The most disastrous within living memory was in 1918–1920 just after World War I when it is estimated to have caused 20 million deaths among 700 million clinical cases worldwide – many more than were killed in the War. The A2-Hong Kong strain influenza epidemic of 1957 was estimated to have caused some 10 million cases in the UK – 1 in 6 of the population and 5000 extra deaths.

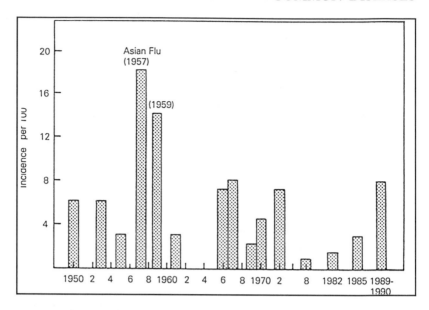

Fig. 3.2—Influenza epidemics 1947–1990 – incidence per 100

Who gets it and when?

Between 1947 and 1990 I recorded 15 notable epidemics of influenza (Figure 3.2).

The extent varied between epidemics with those of 1957–1959 being the most dramatic. Note that these rates represent only those patients who consulted and there must have been many others who were managed by their families alone. The *age distribution* (Figure 3.3) shows that whilst the incidence was highest in children and the middle-aged all ages were affected.

How does it present?

The impact of an extensive influenza epidemic on a community is a near disaster with many persons being infected over a relatively short period of 8–10 weeks.

Generally, the first cases occur in schoolchildren who seem to spread the infection to their families and then to the rest of the population.

The clinical spectrum is broad from subclinical or minimal symptoms to rare deaths within a few hours in overwhelming infections. In children and the elderly, dramatic acute illness is not customary. Young and middle-aged adults tend to go down with

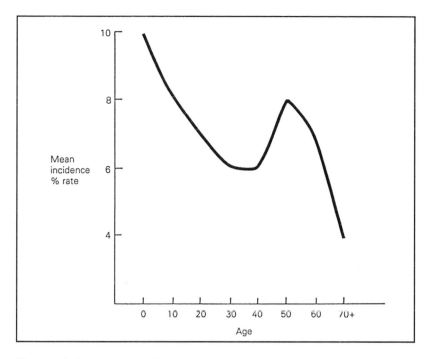

Fig. 3.3—Influenza – age incidence per 100 at risk

dramatic suddenness often pinpointing onset to the hour. In them the onset is with extreme malaise, weakness, aches and pains, headache, eyes aching, fever, cough and nasal obstruction.

What happens?

The *course* in uncomplicated cases is a slow recovery over a few days but there may be a more prolonged period of weeks of lethargy, depression and general physical weakness.

In my own practice the *mortality* from influenza during 1947–1990 was low, 2 per 1000 patients seen and treated.

However, *complications* did occur in just over 10% of cases. Pneumonia and acute bronchitis with prolonged illness and abnormal physical chest signs were most common, with occasional otitis media in children and sinusitis in adults.

Although incidence of influenza was lowest in the elderly they were most prone to complications (Figure 3.4).

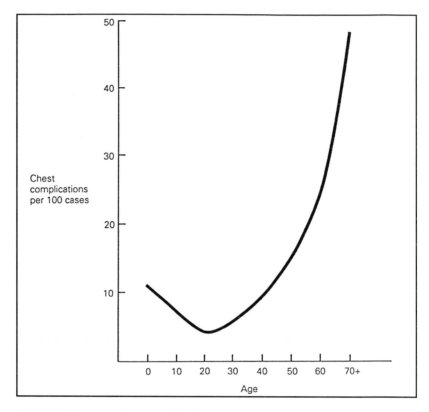

Fig. 3.4—Influenza – chest complications at various ages per 100 cases

The *course* of a *typical influenza epidemic* was of a slow build-up of cases reaching a peak within 2–3 weeks and then gradual decline (Figure 3.5).

It has to be noted that not only are patients affected but also members of the practice team.

What to do?

The most important steps in management are to prepare and organize the practice to meet the epidemic since there is usually a few weeks warning through the media and health departments.

• Produce a protocol for response to demands for care and advice.
• Decide on clinical management.

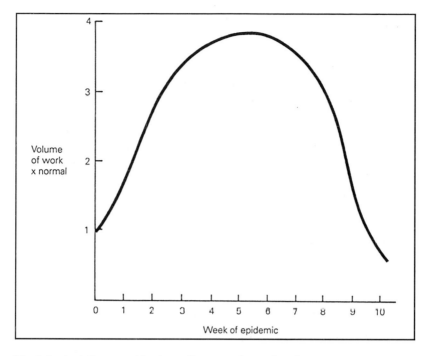

Fig. 3.5—An influenza epidemic – effects on volume of work

- Organize a home visiting rota between doctors and nurses to patients who may require such home visits – most families can cope with suitable advice and support. Decide on what advice is to be given and by whom and how.
- Organize for social and welfare arrangements such as sickness certification, home care of the elderly and disabled.

The *clinical management* will be in two parts – general and specific.

General

Advice on relief of symptoms with analgesics, hot drinks, etc. and instructions on appearances of possible complications.

Specific

Antibiotic protocols for chest complications.
Prophylactic antibiotics are not advisable in general but may be for known individuals.

Prevention

There is uncertainty and controversy over preventive immunization against influenza.

In theory, certain vulnerable groups – elderly and chronic invalids and practice staff members – are recommended for vaccination.

In practice this has to be an extensive and expensive annual exercise, with vaccines that are not necessarily likely to be effective, and also the unpredictability of an epidemic.

Note that major epidemics are likely only every 10 years.

Each practice has to decide its own policy on annual immunization against influenza.

Influenza-like illness

What is it?

A useful label for acute upper respiratory infections that are more disabling than common colds and with more systemic symptoms. Presumably they are caused by various viruses but with no correlations with clinical features.

Who gets it and when?

It is likely that there will be 50 cases per 2000 or 250 per 10 000 in a year.

The age incidence is similar to that of other common upper respiratory infections – (Figure 3.1) with highest rates in children and then progressive decline (RCGP Occasional Paper 53, 1991, on 'Annual & Seasonal Variation in the Incidence of Common Diseases'.)

What happens?

The course is for a natural recovery within 7–10 days and with few complications.

What to do?

Symptomatic measures as noted on pages are all that is required.

Practical points

- Common acute upper respiratory infections are the largest group of common diseases and yet their classification and understanding of causes is unclear.
- Common colds and coughs account for an annual patient consulting rate of 15% but probably most persons are infected every year. Most prevalent in young children. Simple and safe non-specific management is best.
- Epidemic influenza occurs infrequently – major epidemics every 10 years. Caused by specific influenza viruses with continually changing strains and therefore prophylactic immunization is uncertain and has to be given annually.
- Effects of an extensive virulent influenza epidemic can be disastrous on a practice and on a nation.
- Incidence variable but whilst all ages are infected most prevalent in young and middle-aged.
- Complications (pneumonia and bronchitis) most likely in elderly.
- Influenza-like illness is probably merely a common upper respiratory infection with more severe general symptoms. It is not epidemic annually and has no relationship to true epidemic influenza.

CHAPTER 4

THE CATARRHAL CHILD SYNDROME

What is it?

Early experience in general practice/family medicine soon reveals that respiratory disorders are frequent and that within the population it is children in their first 10 years who are most likely to suffer from the various clinical respiratory conditions (Figure 4.1).

In any year about two-thirds of all children in their first decade will consult in a year – a much higher rate than for other disorders (Figure 4.2).

These conditions have a wide clinical spectrum and may present with colds, coughs, earache, sore throat, wheezy chests and general misery and sub-health.

They are important because they are so frequent and take up much consulting time, but also because they lead to much ill health in children and anxiety for parents and school teachers because of absences, because they are not easy to treat since responses are slow and recurrences frequent and because they may lead to pulmonary disabilities in adult life.

In spite of their frequency the causes are uncertain and unproven. It is assumed that they are infections caused by *viruses* but the specific pathogens are rarely isolated; *bacteria* may be responsible

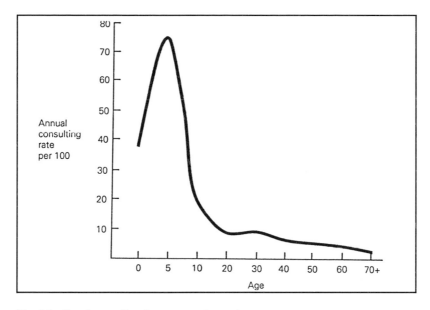

Fig. 4.1—Respiratory disorders – annual prevalence

for a minority of ear, throat and chest infections but again they are isolated in a minority of cases. Whilst *allergy* has been put forward as a possibility there is no reliable evidence for this. Undoubtedly some children and some families appear to suffer more frequently and more seriously than others and therefore it is likely that there may be underlying *social, familial* and *genetic* factors.

Considering the wellnigh inevitability of children suffering from variants of one syndrome and the fact that they appear to 'outgrow' it and gradually cease to suffer from it after the age of 7 to 8 it is likely to be a natural response of an *immature immunological system* to various external environmental pathogens, pollutants and irritants and that given time a natural immunity develops.

Because of the broad nature and wide spectrum of the syndrome it is appropriate that a homely title should be given – '*the catarrhal child syndrome*'.

Who gets it and when?

A feature of all clinical components of the syndrome is the age prevalence distribution (Figure 4.3).

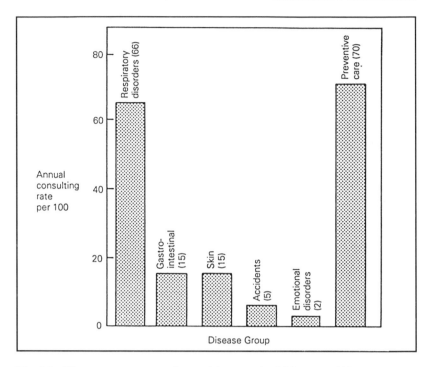

Fig. 4.2—Disease groups – annual consulting rates in children, per 100

It occurs all through childhood but the highest prevalence is between 3 and 8 years possibly because this is the time when children begin to mix more widely socially with other children and adults and particularly when they start school (at 3 to 5). Note that as many as 80% of children consult at 5 to 6 years. Note also the decline in prevalence after age of 7 to 8.

This represents a pattern of natural history (see page 12, Chapter 1) that has to be understood in management.

How does it present?

Because of non-correlation between specific pathogens and specific clinical entities classification has to be on practical clinical features.

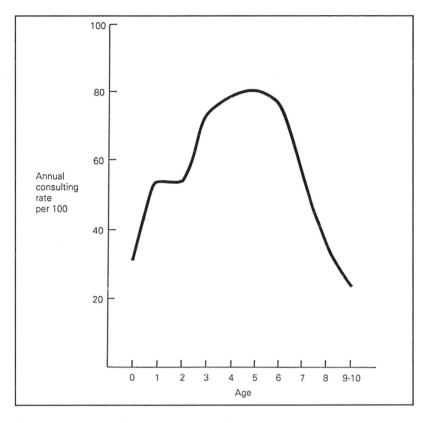

Fig. 4.3—Catarrhal children – annual consulting rates

Four main clinical groups can be separated in these children:

- coughs, colds and catarrh (CCC)
- earaches, deafness and discharge (acute otitis media and glue ear)
- sore throats, enlarged lympth nodes and croup (tonsillitis, laryngitis)
- wheezy chests and other abnormal chest signs (bronchitis, pneumonia, asthma)

(These are discussed in more detail in Chapters 2, 5, 6, 8–10.)

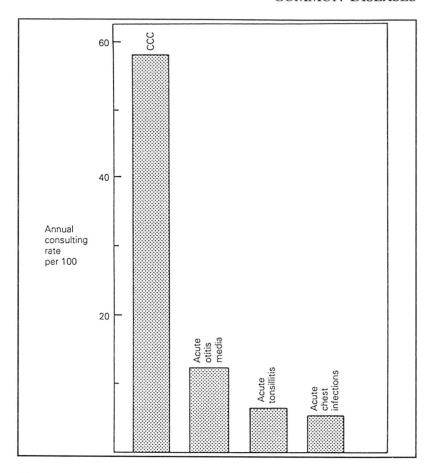

Fig. 4.4—Catarrhal children – clinical groups

Here some general comments are appropriate.

Coughs, colds, catarrh (CCC)

This is the largest group. It comprises blocked nose with discharge and cough that is worse at night plus varying degrees of sub-health, not eating, unhappiness and fractiousness plus considerable anxiety among parents and grandparents.

These features may occur as attacks or they may persist over many weeks. They occur most frequently in the winter months and tend to appear within a few weeks of return to school after summer holidays. Parents tend to consult more with first children probably because of their own inexperience and uncertainty and among parents mothers are more likely than fathers to suffer from similar CCC features.

Earache, deafness and discharge (see also Chapter 5)

Because the middle ear communicates with the upper respiratory tract, via the tympanic tube, it is not surprising that otitis media also is frequent in children. Its frequency has not changed over my (J.F.) 45 years in practice but it has become much more benign with fewer instances of discharge and no spread of infection to the mastoids. On the other hand 'glue ear' or 'catarrhal otitis media' appears to have become more notable. Middle ear infections follow the age prevalence pattern of the syndrome with high rates in the first 7–8 years and then a natural decline.

Throat infections (see also Chapter 6)

There is a distinction between *acute tonsillitis* which is relatively uncommon in young children but more so at 5 to 8 years and again in the teens and more generalized sore throat with *pharyngitis*. The specific condition of *acute croup or laryngitis* which occurs in infants (6 months – 2¼ years), with classical barking cough at night and difficulty in breathing, is not frequent and *acute epiglottitis* is very rare (I have seen one case in 45 years) but potentially life threatening.

Acute chest infections (see also Chapter 8)

These are a part of the syndrome and three clinical forms are recognizable:

- *Acute wheezy chests* with persistent distressing cough, some breathing difficulty and characteristically wheezy sounds on both sides of the chest. It is debatable whether these should be labelled as 'asthma' or 'acute bronchitis'. Whatever the label the majority of such susceptible children cease their attacks after 8–10 years of age and few continue wheezing in adult life.
- *Diffuse moist signs* (acute bronchitis) – these affect infants (0–3 years) who present with respiratory distress and generalized moist rales throughout the lungs and are potentially dangerous.
- *Localized chest signs* (pneumonia) usually in a child with a persistent cough and malaise and on examination a localized area of moist rales or rhondhi is present. This denotes a localized area of pneumonia or peumonitis.

What happens?

As noted the syndrome has a particular pattern of natural history. It is the example of a condition that is prevalent in childhood and which ceases naturally. An explanation has been given (page 49) suggesting a natural process of a build-up of immunity.

Whatever the explanation the implications are of importance to management.

- A reassuring explanation of the course can be given to parents emphasizing the likelihood of 'growing out' without long-term harmful effects.
- Treatment should be realistic and less than drastic and radical knowing the likely good natural outcome, avoiding potentially dangerous surgery or medication.

What to do?

Successful sensitive and sensible management requires a systematic personal plan by each physician based on a clear understanding of the nature and likely course and outcome of the syndrome.

To repeat:

- Specific causes are uncertain and there is no correlation between likely pathogens and clinical features.
- It is a wellnigh inevitable 'normal-abnormality' of childhood.
- It follows a course towards a natural 'cure' with good outcome and few is any permanent ill-effects.

The *basic ingredients* for good care are:

- good rapport with and support of the parents;
- relief of symptoms where possible;
- discrimination in use of 'cures' such as surgery and drugs.

Assessment and diagnosis

Whilst the syndrome is so common this must not blind the physician to miss rarer possibilities for other conditions with similar clinical features:

- *Fibrocystic disease* is the most frequent genetic disorder with liability to serious infections of lungs, nasal polypi, retarded growth and possible respiratory and cardiac failure.
- *Immune deficiency* states either natural or secondary to treatment with chemotherapy lead to liability to serious respiratory infections.
- *Bronchiectasis* now is rare but presents with persistent chronic pulmonary infection.
- *Allergy* may be a factor in hypersensitive children with a family history of asthma or hay fever.
- *Foreign bodies in nose or tracheo-bronchial passages* should be remembered as possible causes of unilateral bloodstained or purulent nasal discharge or sudden and persistent cough and local wheezing.
- *Sinus infections* are rare in children apart from those with fibrocystic disease.

Investigations

In general there are no indications for 'routine' investigations.

Tests that attempt to isolate possible specific pathogens are not really helpful in clinical practice.

The only situation where it is important to know the causal organisms is in children with chronic pulmonary infections in fibrocystic disease.

Throat swabs to isolate *Streptococcus pyogenes* are advocated by some but unless they provide rapid results (within minutes) they do not help to decide on use of antibiotics.

Blood tests are only of practical value when glandular fever (IM) (see Chapter 7) or some rare blood disorder is suspected.

Chest X-rays are indicated when abnormal clinical chest signs persist or in children with recurring serious chest infections or when an inhaled foreign body is suspected. X-rays of nasal sinuses are rarely helpful.

Rapport–support

Probably the most important part in effective management is to establish good relations with the parents of the child and spend time, at the very beginning of the relationship, to explain and inform on the likely nature, course and outcome and to emphasize the facts that there will be a period of recurring problems over 3–4 years but that after age 7–8, or perhaps sooner, the child will outgrow the condition and that serious after-effects are rare. That there is much that can be done to relieve symptoms but that 'cures' are not possible and that strong measures such as frequent use of drugs such as antibiotics or surgical operations should be used with caution.

The mother should be reassured and invited to seek help from the practice team whenever she feels the need. In this way early anxieties can be relieved and self confidence built up.

General relief

Symptomatic measures are important but of limited value. Parents must feel that the physician is concerned enough to recommend relief if not cure. Merely stating that 'there is nothing to be done' is a certain way to lead to poor rapport and relations.

Homely self-care remedies should be encouraged such as hot drinks, analgesics, demulcent linctuses, possibly anti-histaminic preparations for their incidental sedative effects at night, possibly nasal vasoconstrictors but these are unpopular with children.

Specific measures

Antibiotics

Most of the common respiratory infections in children do not require antibiotics, although often the physician is tempted to prescribe them as a 'line of least resistance' and probably they act as placebos rather than as specifics.

There are few real indications – the causal organisms are unlikely to be antibiotic-sensitive, the risk of producing resistant strains is significant, the benefits are no greater than in controls and their use tends to lead to the notions in parents that the conditions are serious and dangerous and that each episode requires the drugs.

In my own practice I find it necessary to prescribe antibiotics in:

- ¼ of sore throats
- ⅓ of earaches
- ½ of chest infections

The indications for their use must be based on:

- age – more so in infants and young children with chest and ear infections
- past history of serious infections
- social circumstances – more in deprived children

- the illness – its presenting severity, disturbance and duration.

Surgery (see also Chapters 5 and 6)

In appropriate cases removal of chronic infected tonsils and enlarged adenoids is beneficial as is drainage of middle ear and insertion of grommets in glue ears.

There is uncertainty over the indications and uncertainty over the rates and it is advisable to have a more conservative than liberal approach.

Practical points

- Catarrhal child syndrome is a useful and practical term for a collection of common respiratory infections of childhood.
- It comprises coughs, colds and catarrh; middle ear infections; throat infections; acute wheezy chests, bronchitis and pneumonia.
- Almost all children suffer from one or more of the variants in their first decade and this probably represents reactions of an immature immunological system to atmospheric pathogens, irritants and pollutants.
- Characteristic pattern of natural history with prevalence at 3–8 years followed by natural 'cure'.
- Management must be based on good rapport and support of the anxious parents of young children suffering from recurrent respiratory problems and sub-health.
- Symptomatic relief with advice on simple self-care measures.
- Selective, sensible and sensitive use of antibiotics and surgery.
- Antibiotics indicated only in a minority of these common infections and tonsillectomy, adenoidectomy and myringotomy and grommets also indicated in a minority.

CHAPTER 5

ACUTE OTITIS MEDIA

Acute otitis media is one of the diseases of general practice/family medicine scarcely seen by specialists.

Apart from its high prevalence it is important because of the suffering and discomfort it causes among young children, often recurring over some years, the disturbances and anxieties caused to parents and to possible effects such as associated loss of hearing, although temporary, which may lead to behavioural upsets and difficulties in learning.

It provides challenges to care in managing the disease, the child and the parents.

What is it?

Acute otitis media is part of the catarrhal child syndrome (Chapter 4). It is associated with coughs, colds and catarrh and has a similar age prevalence and course.

Basically it is an inflammation of the middle ear with accompanying painful swelling of the lining mucosa, exudation of mucosa or purulent fluid. The drum is affected becoming red and swollen and this appearance is the prominent diagnostic sign.

The reason for the high prevalence of acute otitis media in young children is said to be the relatively short Eustachian (tympanic) tube also set at a less acute angle than in adults and this facilitates spread of organisms from the oropharynx into the middle ear.

The *pathogens* are various. Although it is believed that specific bacteria, *Haemophilus influenzae* and pneumococci predominate, when attempts have been made to isolate them from the middle ear (by aspiration) or throat swabs, they are detected in a minority of cases. It is postulated that the remainder are caused by 'viruses' but no specific viruses have been isolated.

These observations are important in deciding on specific treatment – if specific bacteria cannot be blamed for all attacks of acute otitis media, then why should all attacks be treated with antibiotics? (see page 49).

Glue ear is also a part of the catarrhal child syndrome. It is a relatively new label for what used to be called 'catarrhal otitis'. It has become more prominent, but not necessarily more prevalent, because of popularity of the new surgical measures of myringotomy, suction and insertion of grommets.

Glue ear is the accumulation of thick sticky mucus in the middle ear which does not escape along the Eustachian tube and which may take too long a time to absorb naturally.

Its relation to acute otitis media is unclear because it does not always follow an acute attack, it may occur in some children spontaneously and is liable to recur (see also pages 64).

Chronic otitis media is quite a distinct disease from acute otitis media. It is usually a condition of adults, of uncertain cause, with chronic infection that may destroy the ossicles and spread to mastoid, labyrinth and intracranial structures.

Who gets it and when?

The age prevalence of acute otitis media is that of other components of the catarrhal child syndrome (page 47). It occurs throughout the first decade of life, during infancy and pre-school years but the peak is between 4 and 8 years. Then it becomes uncommon and is rare in adults. Appreciation of this natural pattern is important in management. Acute otitis media is one of the conditions which children 'outgrow' naturally and treatment should be so tailored. The explanation for this course may be that it is, as other parts of the syndrome, related to establishment of a natural immunity and resistance and to anatomical changes with growth in the middle ear and Eustachian tube.

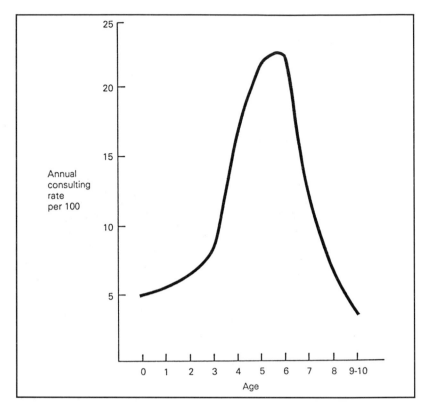

Fig. 5.1—Acute otitis media – annual consulting rates

How does it present?

The clinical presentations differ with different ages. In *infancy*, acute otitis media usually presents as an acutely ill baby, febrile and screaming and obviously in pain, but at this age there is no localization possible. There may be vomiting and rarely a febrile convulsion.

Diagnosis is made by observing a red drum, or drums. In a distressed baby and with anxious parents a good sight of the drums may not be easy and simple!

In *childhood* the most common presentation is *earache* which may be severe–distressing. The onset often is at night and is a frequent reason for a home visit or advice.

The appearance is a red drum, but the examination may be hampered by wax, when diagnosis has to be presumptive.

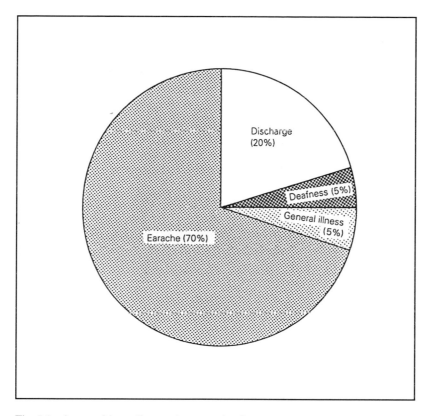

Fig. 5.2—Acute otitis media – main presenting features

Discharge through the ear drum now is less frequent than in the past (20–30 years ago).

Deafness is unusual as the initial presentation but accompanies the acute attack with swelling of the drum and accumulation of exudate.

Glue ear presents as a deaf child, often with no preceding history of earache. The supposed appearance of fluid in the middle ear is difficult to detect with the common auriscope and diagnosis is on the history from the mother.

What happens?

Acute otitis media now is a benign condition of childhood which, as noted, causes considerable distress. This is different from 50 years ago when, for various reasons such as high virulence of streptococci, social factors such as poor nutrition and housing and no antibiotics, complications occurred, such as mastoiditis, intra-cranial sepsis, septicaemia and even death.

In the *typical case* with earache, malaise and fever, and with a red drum, the usual course is for the acute phase to last a couple of days and then resolve naturally – without antibiotics. However, the drum will remain dull, red or pink for 2–3 weeks before returning to normal. Deafness, likewise, may take 2–3 weeks to resolve.

Discharge, now, is unusual but when it occurs it is accompanied by relief of pain. Blood stained and mucopurulent at first it becomes mucoid and tends to cease within a week. Swabs do not usually grow any specific pathogens.

Recurrent attacks are common but cease after the age of 7–8.

Serious complications, as noted, now are very rare but nevertheless the possibility of *mastoiditis* should be remembered with continuing illness, possibly with discharge and tenderness over the mastoid process. The possibility of *cerebral abscess or meningitis* is extremely rare but again has to be remembered.

The *course and outcome* may be related to certain risk factors. Problems such as slow resolution, severity of attacks and as indications for antibiotics are: previous or recurring attacks, a family history of ear troubles, lower social class and associated ear discharge.

What to do?

To recap. Acute otitis media now is a benign disease but highly prevalent, with about one half of all children suffering one or more episodes during their first 10 years. It is presumably infective, but specific bacterial pathogens are found (when tested for) in a minority of cases. Recurrences are frequent but the course is that of a natural decline and cessation of attacks after the age of 7–8.

The components of care must be:

- relief of pain
- support of parents
- indications for antibiotics
- follow-up until drum and hearing are normal
- indications for referral to a specialist.

Relief of pain

The first priority must be relief of pain and distress with analgesics of sufficient strength and frequency. Each practitioner will have his/her routine but the dose should be sufficient to control the pain.

Ear drops or nasal drops do not appear to have any benefits and merely add to the child's discomfort.

Parental support

In all childhood diseases it is essential to spend time to explain to parents the nature of the condition, the likely course and outcome and proposed management and encourage questions.

It is also part of good care to assure availability and accessibility and to offer advice as and when felt necessary.

Antibiotics

The use of antibiotics in acute otitis media is debatable and practitioners range widely in usage rates. Fortunately most antibiotics appear free from serious side-effects for the child but there are risks from development of antibiotic resistant strains of organisms. Antibiotics are more expensive than analgesics and routine usage tends to create the impression among parents that all infections of childhood require antibiotics.

A *selective and discriminating* policy should be set out by each practitioner. This is not easy, but a challenge to good practice.

Indications

My personal approach is to endeavour to avoid routine use of antibiotics but to consider them in the following situations.

- In *severe illness*. I must admit to prescribing them for a severely ill toxic and febrile child, with severe pain and who appears 'really sick'. However, it is a common experience for such severely distressed children to be remarkably better the next day!
- A *past history* of recurrent attacks makes one more likely to use antibiotics. Here there is a case for allowing the parents to have a supply at home and commence treatment at onset of attack. On occasions in a few children with very frequent attacks I have used small dose continuous antibiotics as a preventive measure.
- *Ear discharge* that persists for more than a few days may be an indication.
- *Social and family history* – I would be more likely to consider antibiotics in children from poor home backgrounds and with a family history of ear disease in parents or siblings.

Which antibiotic?

The choice is personal to the physician. At present the most popular are oral amoxycillin or ampicillin with erythromycin for penicillin-sensitivity. However, there are many other choices. The duration of therapy is controversial. Short 3-day courses appear as effective as 5 or 7 days.

Glue ear

The dilemma for the generalist is whether to wait for natural resolution or to refer to a specialist for possible surgery? Again, this is a situation requiring the 'art of care' rather than its science.

On the one hand the condition is certain to resolve given time – but how long? On the other hand if there are effects on communication, learning and behaviour then actions tend to be demanded by parents.

Follow-up

Whatever treatment is given it is important that children who have suffered an attack of acute otitis media be followed up and checked until the condition and function have returned to normal. Therefore, the child should be seen periodically over a few weeks until the drum and hearing are normal.

In a normal practice objective hearing tests in children are impractical and reliance has to be on the parents' opinions. Persisting deafness may be an indication for specialist advice.

Referral to a specialist

Acute otitis media is a condition of primary care. The help of a specialist is indicated for possible after-effects or unusual course and complications.

Whatever the indications it is important that the referring physician knows well his specialist colleague and vice versa. It is important that both understand why the referral is being made and with what expectations for all concerned!

- *For reassurance of parents*: Recurrent attacks and slow resolution are natural worries for parents and these may not be resolved by the generalist's explanation and support. When referral is made it should be clearly stated by the referrer why it is being made and what is expected from the specialist!

- *For possible surgery*: The most usual reason for referral now is for 'glue ear' and possible *suction and insertion of grommets*. Another possibility is *removal of adenoids* on the supposition that enlargement interferes with drainage from the Eustachian tube.

  It has to be re-emphasised that the actions depend on the views and customs of the specialist. There are radical and conservative surgeons – the outcomes of their treatments appear similar!

Practical points

- Acute otitis media is part of the catarrhal child syndrome.
- One-half of all children will suffer one or more attacks.
- Pathogenic organisms are isolated from a minority of cases; it is assumed that others are caused by 'viruses' but the condition may also occur as an inflammatory process without infection.
- The natural history is for appreciable prevalence in infancy and early childhood with peak at 4–8 years and then a natural decline. Rare in adults.
- Clinical presentations are as an unhappy screaming febrile infant; as a child with earache; or with ear discharge or deafness. Diagnosis is by viewing a red drum but this is not always easy.
- Acute otitis media now is a benign condition with few complications. It is a recurring condition in some children.
- Most cases will settle naturally within a couple of days.
- Management must be based on understanding of natural course and outcome.
- Principles of treatment are:
  relief of pain
  support of parents
  selective use of antibiotics
  follow-up until return to normal
  discriminating referral to specialist for possible surgery for glue ear with suction and grommets and/or adenoidectomy.
- Glue ear is a new label for an old condition. It may be distinct from acute otitis media. It causes deafness with difficulties in communication, learning and behaviour. Although it tends to resolve naturally it may require surgical drainage.

CHAPTER 6

ACUTE THROAT INFECTIONS

What are they?

Acute throat infections are a frequent cause of ill health. They comprise a collection of disorders whose prominent clinical features are sore throat and variable degrees of accompanying general ill health.

Diagnostic labels are unhelpful because similar clinical appearances may be produced by various causal agents, and vice versa.

However, it is customary to distinguish between 'tonsillitis', 'pharyngitis' and 'laryngitis' but such terms, whilst useful as entries on sickness certificates, are unhelpful in deciding on aetiology and logical therapy.

The *causes* of acute throat infections may be bacterial or viral and there may be some specific underlying diseases that lead to them.

The most likely pathogenic bacteria are *Streptococcus pyogenes*, but attempts to isolate the organism are successful only in about 40% of all throats. Note that now *diphtheria* is unknown in developed countries, but 50 years ago it was a significant cause of death.

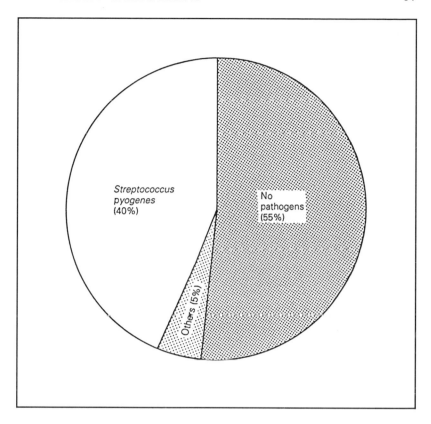

Fig. 6.1—Acute tonsillitis – causes

No specific pathogens can be detected in 55% and possibly the remaining 5% are associated with glandular fever (IM) and rarely with immunodeficient conditions, such as leukaemia, agranulocytosis, HIV infections or following chemotherapy for malignancies. A *local malignancy* is very rare, but should be considered in persistent 'sore throat' in an elderly person, particularly when associated with hoarseness and/or dysphagia. It may arise from a tonsil, pharynx or larynx.

In practice, then, less than one-half are caused by common known bacteria and the remainder probably caused by indeterminate viruses associated with other common upper respiratory infections.

Who gets them and when?

A practice with 2000 patients can expect 120 acute throat infections a year. Of these, 3 will be part of glandular fever (IM) and 1 or 2

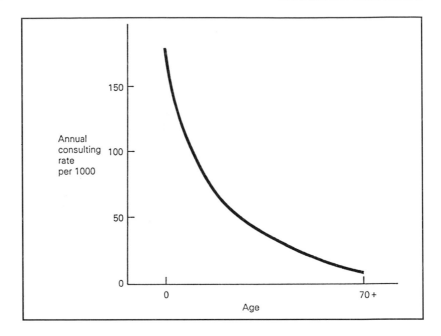

Fig. 6.2—Acute tonsillitis – annual consulting rates (0–70 years)

'scarlet fever'. Associations with immunodeficient state may occur once every 5–10 years only.

The age distributions are characteristic and must be appreciated. Figure 6.2 shows that in the population as a whole acute throat infections occur predominantly in children and young adults.

When age prevalence rates are examined in detail for the 0–25 age groups, two peaks of prevalence are evident:

- between 5 and 10 years
- in 15–25 age group.

Sore throats are rare in infants and young children and in the elderly.

Reasons for these observations must be hypothetical. The 5–10 year peak probably is part of the catarrhal child syndrome (Chapter 4). The 15–25 years peak probably is related also to some immunological changes that seem to make young adults liable to suffer from EBV (Epstein-Barr virus) infections causing clinical glandular fever (IM) and possibly also subclinical infections.

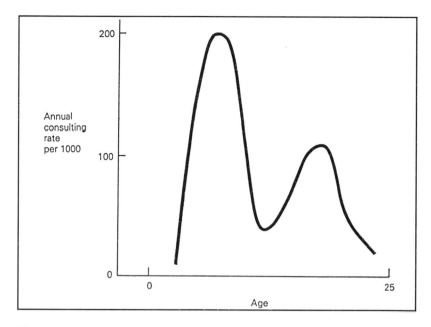

Fig. 6.3—Acute tonsillitis – annual consulting rates (0–25 years)

Seasonally acute throat infections are most prevalent in late winter (February–March) and early winter (November–December), but sometimes collections of cases occur during hot dry summer months.

How do they present?

Sore throat of a few days duration is the presenting symptom. It may be accompanied by a cold or cough, but pain on swallowing is the prominent feature.

There is a variable degree of *general malaise and illness*. High fever and toxicity are more likely with a streptococcal infection.

The appearance of the *fauces* also varies. There may be a generalized redness or more local swelling of the tonsils, perhaps with covering exudate and a pitted follicular look. Beware of a painful swelling of one tonsil, it may be a malignancy. Note that sore throats can occur even in tonsillectomized persons.

Tender and swollen *upper cervical glands* can be felt, particularly in streptococcal infections and glandular fever (IM). A bull-neck appearance was a feature of diphtheria. Also in the past, unilateral discrete swellings of neck glands were caused by tubercle infection.

Note, however, that neck glands are easily palpable in all normal children between 5 and 10 years. A *skin rash* may appear. This may be part of a streptococcal infection ('scarlet fever') or a side effect of treatment with antibiotics, specifically ampicillin in glandular fever (IM) or a more general reaction to penicillin or sulphonamides. A skin rash with sore throat may also be part of a viral infection, such as measles, rubella, adenovirus or Coxsackie viruses.

What happens?

The *normal course* for an acute throat infection is for resolution within a week. Antibiotics may shorten this period by a day or two. The *duration* is longer in glandular fever (IM).

A *prolonged course* must be an indication to reconsider the diagnosis and undertake detailed investigations.

Recurrent attacks are frequent in children and adolescents. An episode of glandular fever (IM) in a teenager is often the beginning of a series of recurrences over a few years that may lead to tonsillectomy as an attempted cure.

Recurrent attacks of sore throat appear to cease after the age of 25 years.

Complications

These may be local or remote.

Local complications

Peritonsillitis or quinsy occurs when infection spreads from tonsillar bed to adjacent tissues leading to marked swelling, oedema and possible abscess formation. Pain is severe, accompanied by trismus, inability to swallow, dribbling of saliva from mouth and toxicity. It is a condition of adults, and I (J.F.) have never seen it in a child under 15 years. It should respond to high doses of intramuscular or intravenous antibiotics.

Rarely, *cervical adenitis* may lead to abscess formation requiring drainage, but as noted, the possibility of tuberculosis or some other rare cause of persistent neck gland swelling should be considered.

Remote complications

These are now rare but possible as results of auto-immune reactions:

- *Acute nephritis* is said to follow streptococcal infections, but in over 40 years only 2 out of 6 cases actually followed a known throat infection.
- *Rheumatic fever* is another possibility. I have seen no cases in over 40 years in my practice in SE England, but it still occurs in N. England and Scotland.
- *Erythema nodosum* can occur 2 or 3 weeks after onset. It may be related to the infection or be a side-effect of the treatment with sulphonamides or antibiotics.

What to do?

The *natural course* of most acute throat infections is for them to resolve within a week or less, but, nevertheless, explanation to the patient, relief of symptoms and possible specific therapy must be considered. It must also be remembered that *specific causes* can be determined in less than one-half of cases even with investigations.

Bearing these points in mind, a logical policy for care has to be made:

- General methods for relief.
- What investigations, if any?
- Indications for and selection of antibiotics.
- Referral to specialist for possible tonsillectomy or other reasons.

General relief measures

Analgesics in adequate dosage should relieve the discomfort. Local measures can include gargles or lozenges. Use of local NSAID gargles or mouthwashes may be effective.

Investigations

Throat swabs to isolate pathogens are of limited practical value. Unless special rapid methods are used within the practice sending the swab to a pathology department will produce a report in 24 hours or more.

Blood tests may be necessary in particular situations when glandular fever (IM) or other blood disorders are considered possibilities.

Urinalysis is indicated in the very rare possibility of renal complications (acute nephritis).

Antibiotics

Indications for antibiotics should be considered on an individual basis and on clinical grounds such as:

- severity of illness – discomfort, toxicity
- for 'local' tonsillitis rather than for 'general' pharyngitis
- previous attacks (recurrences)
- associated with other illness
- complication such as quinsy or large tender cervical glands
- some personal, social or other reason where a quick response is hoped for.

I (J.F.) find I use antibiotics in about one-third of acute throat infections.

Which antibiotic?

Streptococcus pyogenes still is sensitive to penicillin. Therefore, penicillin V (phenoxypenicillin) is recommended by intramuscular or oral routes. For the severely ill, intravenous route (in hospital) may be necessary. Do *not* use ampicillin or amoxycillin as side-effects (rashes) will occur in glandular fever (IM).

For penicillin-sensitive persons, erythromycin is recommended.

Referral to specialist

Persons who suffer from recurrent attacks of tonsillitis should be considered for tonsillectomy. Whilst in time most will cease to suffer attacks, the question arises – how long should one wait?

The most usual situations are:

- a teenager or young adult suffering recurring bouts of localized acute tonsillitis following confirmed glandular fever (IM) some time past
- a child 5–10 years old with recurring sore throats and perhaps earaches as well.

In both situations removal of tonsils, and perhaps adenoids in the second case, should be considered.

Persons with quinsy who do not improve with high doses of antibiotics for 2–3 days should be considered for admission to hospital for more intensive treatment.

Practical points

- Acute throat infections are common in practice, two or three cases per practitioner per week.
- Specific pathogens or causes are discovered in less than one-half of attacks.
- Age prevalence peaks in children at 5–10, and young adults 15–25.
- Sore throat infections are rare in early childhood and in old age.
- Presentations may be as a generalized 'pharyngitis' or local 'tonsillitis'.
- Assessment should be on clinical grounds; investigations should be used with discrimination, i.e. throat swabs and blood.
- Most cases will recover naturally within a week, but recurrences are common.
- Antibiotics are probably necessary only in about one in three cases.
- Penicillin still is first choice antibiotic.
- Tonsillectomy may be necessary for persons with recurring attacks.

CHAPTER 7

GLANDULAR FEVER (INFECTIOUS MONONUCLEOSIS : IM)

What is it?

A clinical syndrome of sore throat, generalized enlarged lymph glands, variable degrees of illness and a specific positive blood test for heterophil antibodies.

It is generally accepted to be a systemic infection with Epstein-Barr virus (EBV) of B-lymphocytes with a reactive response by T-lymphocytes which destroy the EBV.

Predominantly an infection of young adults particularly in closed communities such as colleges, universities and military establishments.

However, clinical evidence for cross-infection is weak. In general practice it is rare to find more than a single case every few months with no history of contact.

Note that similar clinical presentation may occur in cytomegalovirus, HIV (AIDS) and toxoplasma infections.

Note that EBV causes Burkitt's lymphoma in Africa and rarely lymphoma may present as an atypical IM.

Who gets it and when?

It is not a common condition with an annual incidence of 1.5 per 1000 or 3 cases in a practice with 2000 and 15 cases in a group with 10 000 patients.

The *age incidence* (Figure 7.1) is characteristic with highest rates at ages 15–25.

'Epidemics' may be seen as clusters of cases where young adults and teenagers live together and there transmission through saliva ('kissing disease') is postulated.

It is rare in young children and in the elderly, where the syndrome is likely to be due to a more sinister cause such as lymphoma or malignancy of tonsil or oropharynx.

'Familial IM' is not uncommon. There are some families whose siblings go down with IM when each reaches teenage. Since they

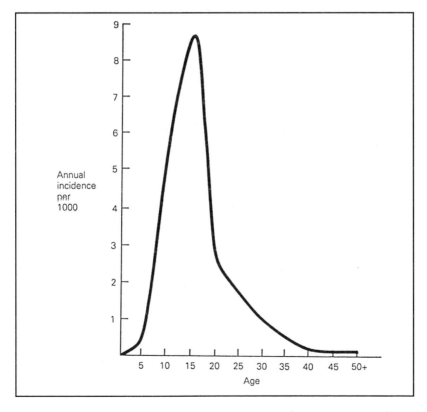

Fig. 7.1—Glandular fever – annual incidence per 1000, 1964–1991

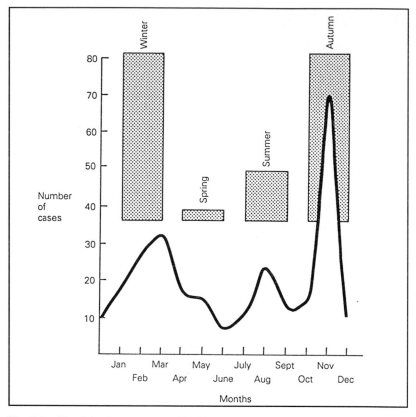

Fig. 7.2—Glandular fever – seasonal incidence, 1964–1981

occur a few years apart it is probable that some genetic immunological trait is the explanation rather than cross-infection.

Seasonal distribution: incidence is highest in winter and autumn.

How does it present?

The usual presentation is of a teenager with:

- Severe sore throat for a week or longer.
- Palpable lymph glands in neck but also in axillae and groin.
- Variable degrees of malaise and toxicity.
- The severity ranges from relatively mild ambulant cases to severely ill, toxis, infected throat and barely able to open mouth.
- It is said that the spleen is enlarged in all cases but this is difficult to detect clinically.

What happens?

Resolution of throat infection usually occurs over a period of 2–3 weeks but enlarged lymph glands may take a few months to return to normal.

Lethargy, weakness–depression may persist for weeks and months and are most distressing for students with curricula to follow. Where tonsils are present *recurrent tonsillitis* may occur at intervals over some years and may lead to tonsillectomy as a cure.

Second attacks are rare but do occur usually in individuals whose first proven episode is at an early age of 10–12 with a confirmed recurrence in late teens or later.

Complications are rare but since the condition is a systemic infection with EBV a range is possible:

- splenomegaly may lead to spontaneous or traumatic rupture of the spleen
- hepatitis is said to occur frequently because of abnormal liver function tests
- skin rashes may be part of the EBV infection or a side-effect of ampicillin which may have been prescribed
- cardiac pericarditis has been reported and myocarditis has been a cause of death
- neurological complications are very rare but include encephalitis, transverse myelitis, cranial nerve palsies and Guillain-Barre syndrome
- renal – nephritis
- lung – interstitial pneumonia
- multiple painful joints
- blood — acute haemolytic anaemia
                — thrombocytopenia
                — agranulocytosis and agammaglobulinaemia.

Fortunately these complications tend to resolve completely in time but supportive management in hospital may be required.

What to do?

Diagnosis

A *high clinical index of suspicion* of IM is required when a teenager or young adult presents with a persistent sore throat, enlarged glands and malaise – particularly when there has been no response to antibiotics, or a rash after ampicillin.

Confirmation is by a confirmatory blood test with 20% or more of atypical mononuclear lymphocytes and positive Paul–Bunnell test or monospot screening test for heterophil antibodies. These tests may not become positive until the second week of the illness, so repeats may be indicated. They remain positive for some months.

Throat swabs may be negative or grow *Streptococcus pyogenes* as a secondary infection.

Management

Once the diagnosis has been confirmed its nature and probable course should be *explained* to the patient noting the slow course and possible delayed return to full health. Although there is no specific treatment for IM, in many cases the severe throat infection is caused by infection with *Streptococcus pyogenes*. Therefore penicillin V should be prescribed orally or by intramuscular injections. Do *not* prescribe ampicillin as this produces a rash. The response to penicillin may be pleasingly effective.

Steroids have been recommended for those severely ill with:

- severe throat infections
- neurological complications
- clinical hepatitis
- interstitial pneumonia
- blood complications.

These patients should be managed in hospital.

Practical points

- IM is a clinical syndrome, affecting teenagers and young adults, with sore throats, palpable lymph glands, positive Paul-Bunnell or monospot tests for abnormal heterophil antibodies.
- The illness ranges from mild and almost sub-clinical to very severely ill with throat infection and remote complications.
- Caused by Epstein-Barr virus.
- Most cases resolve within 2–3 weeks, but sometimes with persistent lethargy and depression.
- Familial IM occurs when siblings are affected when they reach teenage.
- Recurrences can occur.
- Although no specific treatment, penicillin V may help by controlling secondary streptococcal infections. (Do not prescribe ampicillin.)
- Cases requiring steroids for complications should be hospitalized.

CHAPTER 8

ACUTE CHEST INFECTIONS (BRONCHITIS AND PNEUMONIA)

What are they?

The group of conditions loosely labelled as 'acute chest infections' illustrates the profound gulf between the practical realities of the clinical problems and presentations facing the family physician in his work and the rather impractical non-realities of the academic scientists and specialists who classify and postulate on the conditions as seen in their own special and artificial context. The result is confusion and uncertainty. The approach in family practice must be practical and realistic and one that will help the family physician in his approach, assessment and management of these patients.

Acute chest infections are the largest group of major diseases that the family physician encounters. They have a case mortality rate of 3% and present considerable challenges to good care in family practice.

Acute chest infections are a difficult group to categorize and define neatly and precisely. The first problems are uncertainty of diagnosis and aetiological labelling. It is difficult, in fact, to decide when the case is acute for it may well be superimposed on some chronic disorder when there is chest involvement as evidence of pulmonary pathology and when there is actual infection present; and the relationship between clinical features and aetiological causes is often impossible to establish.

What then are these acute chest infections? They represent a definable clinical syndrome with cough, fever, purulent sputum, sometimes breathlessness and chest pain, and often, but not always, abnormal clinical physical signs in the chest and radiographic changes to support these findings.

A working definition is of sudden onset, symptoms of a chest infection and abnormal physical or radiographic signs in the chest.

Names and labels

What are their causes and pathology? Here again there is considerable confusion and uncertainty. It is difficult to translate a precise aetiological and pathological classification of acute chest infections from the laboratories and the hospitals to family practice.

An aetiological classification based on precisely defined bacterial and viral causes is not possible in family practice, because methods of investigation are imprecise and impractical. In a study in my practice (J.F.) when all available investigations were used to make an aetiological diagnosis, such a diagnosis was possible in only one-third of all episodes.

A pathological diagnosis based on morbid anatomy is not very helpful in family practice because it is one based on the pathology of the dead, whereas family practice is the care of the living. Whilst 'pneumonia' and its many varieties and 'bronchitis' are terms in everyday use, they have serious practical limitations. The terms provide no more than useful but vague labels with which to classify cases; they offer little in the understanding of the disease processes of the types of conditions encountered in the field of primary care.

The term 'pneumonitis' is a portmanteau attempt to create a mix of 'pneumonia' and 'bronchitis' suggesting something less severe than pneumonia and not quite a bronchitis. More research is required into the acute chest infections in the primary care field in order to define their nature and patterns and to reconsider their taxonomy.

The following clinical groups of acute chest infections have been found to be practical:

- The *'acute wheezy chest'* where the main features are diffuse and bilateral signs over both sides of the chest. The signs are wheezy rhonchi and interspersed occasional scattered moist rales.
- The case with *'local moist sounds'* where the presenting signs are those of an area of inspiratory moist, coarse or fine crackles, usually at one or other lung base, but occasionally in more than one area.
- *Others* that may occur are cases with a pleural rub, or with consolidation, or with effusion or with signs of collapse of part of a lung. These are a small proportion of all cases.
- For completeness there are the cases of acute chest infection where there are *no abnormal physical signs* but where there are radiographic abnormalities of probable infection.

Causes and causal factors

Some bacteria and viruses are recognized as causes of acute chest infections. The bacteria are pneumococci, *Streptococcus pyogenes*, *Haemophilus influenzae*, staphylococci, tubercle bacilli and *Klebsiella pneumoniae* (Friedlander's bacillus) and viruses such as influenza, para-influenza, respiratory syncytial virus (RSV), *Rickettsia burnetti* (Q fever), psittacosis (ornithosis), measles and other organisms such as *Mycoplasma pneumoniae*.

Such a list is required in order to understand the pathology of acute chest infections and to investigate patients in the hospital setting. It is not very useful in the practical context of primary care, where the causal agents are usually indefinable and are a mixture of pathogens superimposed on individual and social factors. A recent group are opportunistic infections associated with AIDS and other immune-compromised conditions. Here *Pneumocystis carinii* is a frequent cause of pneumonia.

The most likely infecting agents encountered in primary care are a mixture of pneumococci and *Haemophilus influenzae* in association with some viral agent. There are a number of other secondary factors that may be important in the development of the infection.

Chest infections may be secondary to some underlying lung disorder such as malignant or benign neoplasms, chronic bronchitis and emphysema, fibrocystic disease (mucoviscoidosis), bronchial stenosis following old tuberculosis, inhaled foreign bodies, bronchiectasis or some other disease and as noted above, AIDS.

Social factors include poor housing, low nutrition, bad working conditions; personal factors include tobacco smoking, old age or early childhood allergies and underlying allergies; familial factors include an inherent predisposition to chest disease that may be associated with some, at present indefinable, diathesis; a past history of some predisposing disorders such as asthma, chronic bronchitis or sinusitis: all these are factors that will render an individual more likely to suffer from acute chest infections.

Smoking and children

There is a strong association in developed countries between infant respiratory tract infection and parental smoking habits. Strongest association is in the first year of life and the association disappears by 3–4 years of age. Also, there is some evidence that the mother's smoking habits during pregnancy rather than after birth are the more important factor predisposing to bronchitis in infancy.

Who gets them and when?

To repeat, acute chest infections are the largest group of major serious diseases encountered in general practice. They are potentially life-threatening, with a 2–3% case fatality and possibly some permanent damage to the respiratory tract.

Apart from the expected pathological changes and effects of acute infection in the lungs and bronchi, there are other changes that cause problems in management.

If sizeable areas of the lungs are affected and put out of action, then respiratory failure occurs with its triad of carbon dioxide retention, anoxaemia and acidaemia. This is much more likely to happen in persons who already have damaged or old and worn lungs and bronchi. Obstruction to the pulmonary circulation by collapse and occlusion of the small lung blood vessels may lead to the state of right-sided heart failure (cor pulmonale). Each attack of acute infection undoubtedly leads to some more permanent damage to respiratory function and with frequent attacks a permanent state of respiratory failure may result.

The annual prevalence rate is 6–7% which means that there will occur approximately 128 acute chest infections in a practice of 2000 persons. Of these:

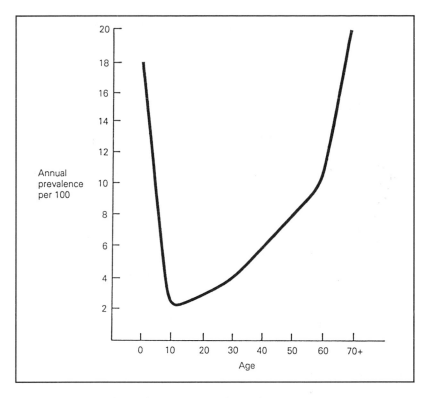

Fig. 8.1—All acute chest infections – age and prevalence

- Acute wheezy chests — 77 (60%)
    (acute bronchitis)
- Localized pneumonia — 39 (30%)
- Pneumonia — 12 (10%)

The male : female distribution of prevalence is 3 : 2. More boys and more elderly men are prone to acute chest infections.

The *age prevalence* of all *chest infections* (Figure 8.1) shows that it is young children and elderly persons who are most susceptible.

There are differences in the three clinical types (Figure 8.2). *Acute wheezy chests (bronchitis)* has the young–old prevalence curve; *localized pneumonias* are most prevalent in children; *major pneumonias* are infrequent and show an increase with age.

How do they present?

It is difficult to match clinical and investigative findings with a probable diagnostic label. Various clinical syndromes may be

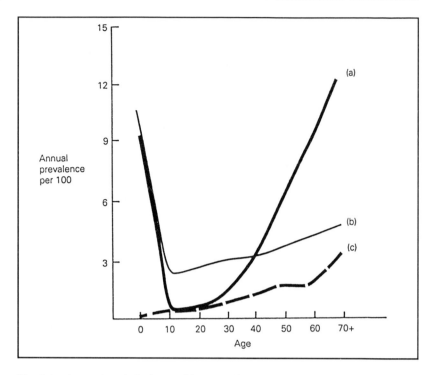

Fig. 8.2—Acute chest infections – (a) acute wheezy chest, (b) localized pneumonias, (c) major pneumonias

caused by a whole range of bacterial and viral organisms with little correlation between them.

The primary physician is faced by a patient with symptoms and signs pointing to a probable acute chest infection. He has to go ahead and manage the situation immediately without waiting for results of diagnostic investigations.

Past history

The previous history of the patient may be of significance. The immediate precedents may be a common upper respiratory infection or influenza or there may be a long history of more chronic chest disease such as chronic bronchitis and emphysema, tuberculosis or recurrent acute chest infections. It is important to make an early assessment of the individual's special liability and vulnerability to chest disease and of his basic state of pulmonary function.

Symptoms

The symptoms of a possible chest infection are cough, sputum, breathlessness, chest pain and general disturbance such as fever, malaise and toxaemia.

The onset may be acute, sudden and devastating with collapse and signs of serious illness. This is the feature of the acute pneumococcal, staphylococcal or influenzal pneumonias, but these are now rare events. Much more frequently the onset is slower and undramatic. The patient presents with a productive cough of a few days' duration, possibly with some breathlessness and vague aches and pains in the chest. He is not apparently very ill and it is on physical examination of the chest or on radiograph that abnormalities are detected.

The cough is productive with mucopurulent yellow, green or brown sputum. Blood staining is not usual and should be a signal for excluding tuberculosis or cancer.

Breathlessness is a feature when there is a lot of wheezing due to bronchial obstruction, when there is considerable underlying pulmonary damage, when there is an associated cardiac failure, or when there is an extensive infection involving large areas of the lungs.

Chest pain may range from a vague ache in the chest overlying the infected areas to a severe sharp pleuritic pain.

The general disturbance is often inconspicuous and most patients are ambulant. Dramatic onset with high fever and severe illness is exceptional.

As a practical summary *the main symptoms* are:

- cough
- sputum
- haemoptysis
- breathlessness
- wheezing
- chest pain

Cough

Commonest symptom due to stimulation of receptors in the large airways triggered by the infection; in viral infections the cough may persist for many weeks.

Sputum

Diagnostic clues to the nature of respiratory tract infection from the appearance of the sputum:

- clear white or grey – chronic bronchitis
- green or yellow – acute infection
- thin and mucoid – viral bronchitis
- 'rusty' sputum – pneumonia
- bloody – lung abscess, bronchiectasis, tuberculosis, aspergilloma – and remember cancer
- thick and sticky – bronchial asthma
- large amounts foul-smelling – bronchiectasis, lung abscess, cystic fibrosis.

Chest pain

The types of chest pain which may be associated with respiratory tract infections include:

- Pleural – sharp stabbing, worse at the side of the chest and worse on inspiration – due to pleurisy with/without underlying pneumonia.
- Mediastinal – raw retrosternal pain worse on inspiration – due to trachea-bronchitis.
- Chest wall pain related to movement and to breathing – can be result of a rib fracture following a bout of prolonged coughing.

Signs

- *Rhonchi (wheezes)* – due to narrowing of the airways by inflammation of the mucosa and associated spasm – this causes the airways to oscillate with respiration like a reed in a musical instrument.
- *Rales (crepitations, crackles)* – due to equalization of intraluminal pressure as the collapsed small airways open up in inspiration. In generalized infection in the lungs gravity causes the rales to be more prominent at the lung bases. If the rales clear with coughing they are unlikely to be of any clinical significance.
- Clinical signs of *consolidation, collapse* and *effusion* are now uncommon.

Specific types of pneumonia

Pneumonia is a general term for infective causes of consolidation of the lungs. In the UK pneumonia causes ten times as many deaths as all other infectious diseases together, and four times as many deaths as asthma in patients under 50 years old.

Although the traditional classification of pneumonia is into lobar pneumonia and bronchopneumonia, it is probably more helpful from the management point of view to look at the particular circumstances and situation in which the pneumonia has occurred and use an alternative grouping:

- community-acquired pneumonia
- hospital-acquired pneumonia
- aspiration pneumonia
- pneumonia associated with immuno-suppressed patients, e.g. AIDS and those on immuno-suppressive drugs for malignant conditions and transplant patients.

Our concern in this book is primarily with the type of pneumonia acquired in the community.

Community-acquired pneumonia

Organisms

- Pneumococci are the commonest cause in the UK
- Other pathogens – *Haemophilus influenzae, Branhamella catarrhalis* (common in chronic bronchitics)
- Virus infections – 10 to 20% of all cases, often complicated by secondary bacterial infection
- *Staphylococcus aureus* – often complicates flu and other viral infections
- *Mycoplasma chlamydia* – uncommon

History

Diagnostic clues:

- Sore throat and upper respiratory symptoms suggest viral or atypical infections.
- Seriously ill within a few hours suggests a pneumococcal or staphylococcal origin.
- Persistent symptoms not responding to penicillins suggest mycoplasma.
- Recent stay in hotel or hospital suggests the possibility of legionella infection.

The *age of the patient* may be helpful in deciding the likely cause of the pneumonia:

- neonates – *H. influenzae*; *Staph. aureus*
- peripartum neonate – *H. influenzae* type B; chlamydia
- pre-school children – pneumococci; respiratory syncytial virus
- school children – pneumococci; mycoplasma
- adults – pneumococci
          atypical infections – Chlamydia
                                   legionella
                                   Q fever
- elderly – *H. influenzae*.

Examination findings in community-acquired pneumonia

- High fever in the young
- Elderly seriously ill, often with no or little fever
- Confusion is common if infection is severe
- *Herpes labialis* common in pneumococcal pneumonia
- Commonest chest signs are inspiratory crackles over the infected area. Signs of consolidation are found in less than 25% of the patients with pneumonia.

Opportunistic infections associated with AIDS

Pneumocystis carinii most important – 85% of all patients with AIDS will have one or more episodes of *P. carinii* pneumonia at some time. Other likely organisms:

- tubercle bacillus
- cytomegalovirus
- pneumococci and *H. influenzae*
- rarely fungal infections, toxoplasma
- herpes simplex, nocardia.

What happens?

The *case fatality* is 2–3%: this means that there are some 60 000 *deaths* from acute chest infections in the UK, or 10% of all deaths. Although only one-half of these are listed as 'pneumonias' the others appear under different labels.

> *Acute chest infections – annual*
> *(practice with 2000 patients)*
> 128   cases
> 20   admitted to hospital
> 2–3   deaths

Where there are no underlying diseases, the recovery rate is good, with clinical resolution within 2 weeks.

In *hospital practice* the overall mortality of community-acquired pneumonia is 5–15%. At-risk factors are age over 60, rapid respiratory rate, low diastolic blood pressure, onset of dysrhythmias and mental confusion.

What to do?

Assessment

Faced with a patient with a probable acute chest infection, the primary physician has to make a number of decisions before embarking on a definite treatment.

- *First,* he has to confirm that it is an acute chest infection. Acute and diffuse wheezing is also a feature of asthma where there is no underlying infection, but there is generally a history of preceding similar attacks. Diffuse crackles and severe breathlessness are features of acute left-sided heart failure. The patient is usually in the late-fifties or upwards, with high blood pressure or some history of myocardial ischaemia.
- *Second,* a decision has to be taken on whether the acute chest infection is primary or secondary in association with some underlying cause. Conditions to be considered and excluded are cancer of the bronchus, tuberculosis and chronic bronchitis, all of which will influence treatment.
- *Third,* an attempt should be made to establish the cause of the infection, but it must be admitted that this is often a forlorn hope because investigations, even of the most intensive nature, do not provide a conclusive answer in the majority of cases. It is certainly important to investigate intensively those that do not respond as expected to treatment, and those who are severely ill.
- *Fourth,* the patient's personal background and family history are important. 'Catarrhal children' between 4 and 8 years of age are likely to suffer attacks of acute chest infections and then to

outgrow them. Asthmatics, chronic bronchitics and heavy smokers are especially liable to recurrent infections. The family history and the home, social and occupational circumstances must all be considered in deciding on the management.

Investigations

Investigations of acute chest infections may be useful, but they are by no means possible or essential in all cases. Certainly, it is always necessary to follow up and investigate the new cases of an acute chest infection in an adult to exclude a possible underlying cause such as cancer of the bronchus or pulmonary tuberculosis, which require special treatment and management. It is less necessary to investigate and re-investigate young children who are passing through the catarrhal phase, or chronic bronchitics, or asthmatics who are well known to suffer recurrent attacks. However, it is necessary to be aware that some of these elderly bronchitics may develop tuberculosis or lung cancer.

Of the investigations, chest radiographs, sputum examinations and respiratory function tests are most often carried out.

- *Chest radiography* should be carried out at some stage during most acute chest infections, but certainly not during each and every attack. The value of chest radiography is to confirm the diagnosis, to localize the lesions, to assess the progress and to exclude other conditions, such as cancer, tuberculosis or other pulmonary pathology.

  For the majority of patients who can be managed at home, chest radiography can be delayed, if the condition is responding to treatment, until the person can attend the local radiography department during convalescence. If there has been little or no progress then a domiciliary chest radiograph can be arranged with the local radiologist. In most instances reasonable films can be obtained with modern portable machines.

- *Sputum examination* for organisms is carried out almost routinely by some physicians, but the tests have strict limitations. Appearance of the sputum is not necessarily related to the bacteriological findings. Purulent-looking sputum, yellow or green in colour, often grows no pathogenic organisms on culture or none are seen on direct examination. In less than a quarter of instances have bacteriological examinations of sputum been useful to me in suggesting possible definitive causation. Examination for viruses has little practical application in everyday practice.

- *Respiratory function tests* are useful in assessing the functional progress of patients following acute chest infections. In particular, such tests are useful in patients with underlying chronic conditions, such as asthma and chronic bronchitis. The simpler the test the better, and the Peak Flow Meter or the Vitalograph are such tests that can be used in any practice.
- *Blood investigations* for general and specific evidence of infection are helpful only on rare occasions, and are not required as routine procedures.

Investigations in patients treated at home

Chest X-ray may be worth considering in the convalescent phase to exclude any serious underlying cause of the pneumonia, especially in a patient who has not had any lung trouble before. *If recovery is unduly slow*, then:

- a chest X-ray is mandatory to look especially for underlying malignancy
- do serological tests for atypical organisms and for viral infections
- test for TB
- test for AIDS if the patient's lifestyle suggests this as a possibility.

Management

Acute chest infections are conditions of primary care, and in J.F.'s practice less than 1 in 10 are referred to the specialists or admitted to hospital.

Having made the diagnosis of an acute chest infection, the first decisions to be made by the physician are whether the patient can be treated by the primary physician at home or in his own hospital unit, or does he require intensive specialist care? If the patient is to remain under the care of the primary physician, what specific and general management is necessary?

Home or hospital?

The decision on home or hospital will depend on individual circumstances. It will depend on the severity of the illness. Most patients with acute chest infections are not usually desperately ill, but some are, and should be in a hospital unit with intensive care facilities. Management will depend on the home facilities, on the type of home and on who is available to nurse the patient. It will depend on the wishes of the patient and the family. It will depend on the attitude of the physician and whether he feels able and prepared to supervise the treatment and management at home or at hospital.

Antibiotics

Specific treatment is concerned with the choice of antibiotic. Response to antibiotics should be evident within two days, with general improvement and some resolution of chest signs. The chest signs, however, may take a few weeks to clear completely in spite of the patient feeling almost completely recovered. It is not necessary to continue antibiotics until all abnormal chest signs have cleared – a period of 7–14 days should be long enough. The patient must be followed up until abnormal signs clear.

There are some cases where antibiotics may not be necessary. Some children suffer recurring chest infections over a few years, and during these bouts they are reasonably well in themselves. It is most important to be guided by the child's general state rather than to be influenced by the physical signs in the chest. If the child is well, then antibiotics can reasonably be withheld. The same reasoning applies to adults with recurring bouts of acute or chronic bronchitis. Many such bouts will settle without antibiotics.

Where antibiotics are considered necessary, the majority of the patients will respond to amoxycillin, which should be the first-line treatment: this should be effective, particularly in pneumococcal and *Haemophilus influenzae* infections.

Second-line treatment includes erythromycin and co-trimoxazole.

For pneumonia occurring during a influenza epidemic, the best drugs are:

- *Co-amoxyclav* – a mixture of amoxycillin with the beta-lactamase inhibitor, clavulanic acid (beta-lactamase produced by bacteria causes penicillin resistance)
- *Flucloxacillin*

Supportive measures

Some patients with acute chest infections have other serious associated disorders; therefore, it may be necessary to treat airways obstruction in asthmatics and chronic bronchitics (see Chapters 9 and 10) and to manage cardiac failure (see Chapter 16).

If oxygen therapy is considered necessary for these acute cases, then this should be an indication for hospitalization.

Bed rest should be minimal and ambulation should be encouraged as soon as feasible.

There is a group of vulnerable individuals who have to be defined and followed up and supported almost continually – those who are liable to recurrent attacks of acute chest infections.

Within this group are:

- some catarrhal children between 3 and 8 years of age;
- some asthmatics in whom acute episodes are associated with chest infections;
- chronic bronchitics and the emphysematous with a defective bronchial tract and diminished respiratory function;
- a mixed bag of patients with a history of past chest illnesses such as tuberculosis, pulmonary fibrosis, those who have undergone chest surgery, and those with certain pulmonary allergies.

These should be seen regularly. Their respiratory function should be tested and they should be given a supply of antibiotics of proven value to them to be taken at the earliest stages of an acute chest infection.

Practical points

- Acute chest infection is the largest group of potentially life-threatening diseases in family practice.
- The annual prevalence in a population of 2000 will be 128:

'acute wheezy chests' (bronchitis)	77
'localized moist sounds' (pneumonia-pneumonitis)	39
'others' (serious pneumonia)	12

- Difficulties face the family physician in endeavouring to relate the clinical features to likely aetiology and pathology.
- Further difficulties result from the fact that many acute chest infections occur in already abnormal lungs, such as asthma and other allergies, chronic bronchitis, bronchial neoplasm, bronchiectasis, occupational lung diseases and fibrocystic disease – therefore, there are double pathologies to consider. Also always consider AIDS.
- Acute chest infections are also affected by factors such as age and sex, occupation, personal habits such as smoking, family history and social class.
- Three clinical presentations are definable (as above):
  acute wheezy chests;
  localized moist sounds;
  signs of consolidation, collapse, effusion or pleurisy.
- Assessment and management are based on clinical features; selective investigations will be necessary in few situations, but any unusual case has to be comprehensively investigated and followed up.
- Antibiotics will be used in most acute chest infections, but are not always required.
- Consider age of the patient in choice of antibiotic – this gives a clue to likely causal organisms.
- Ampicillin or amoxycillin are first choices and then co-trimoxazole or erythromycin.

CHAPTER 9

CHRONIC BRONCHITIS

What is it?

Chronic bronchitis is a term that has been in use for almost 200 years, but only recently has come to mean something more specific and definitive than a persistent productive cough with variable degrees of respiratory deficiency. Yet even now its definition and interpretation create problems and difficulties, particularly when comparisons between different nations and geographical situations are attempted. For, closely associated with chronic bronchitis, is the condition of emphysema, whose main features are abnormally large air spaces in the lungs created through confluence and disappearance of normal lung tissue and leading to loss of pulmonary functional area and respiratory deficiency. The association between chronic bronchitis and emphysema is uncertain and since the aetiology of emphysema is even less well understood than that of chronic bronchitis it is difficult to be more definite about it.

Yet further confusion is created in North America, especially with the apparently high frequency of the diagnosis of 'sinusitis', a condition whose symptoms of productive cough, associated with some nasal catarrh and obstruction, are very similar to those of chronic bronchitis elsewhere.

Chronic bronchitis, then, may mean different things to different physicians and it is important to have some clear and definable understanding of the condition.

95

Chronic bronchitis is *defined* as 'a productive cough occurring on most days for at least 3 months in the year in at least 2 consecutive years'.

In considering its natural history a distinction should be made between chronic mucus hypersecretion (chronic bronchitis) and actual airway obstruction. Chronic mucus hypersecretion is common in smokers, and is the result of pathological changes in the central airways; it is not usually associated with the development of airway obstruction and improves when smoking stops. If airway obstruction does develop, it occurs in the peripheral airways, is not reversible on stopping smoking and often leads to progressive disability and ultimately early death.

The obstructive type of chronic bronchitis is often associated with emphysema, which may be defined as a dilatation and destruction of the terminal air sacs, the alveoli. In practice it is very difficult to separate the contribution of small airway obstruction and the emphysema to the patient's disability.

The *pathological features* of *chronic bronchitis* correspond to the three clinical components:

- excessive mucus production
- recurrent infection
- narrowing of the small airways.

The development of *emphysema* particularly in smokers is due to:

- excessive production of macrophages induced by smoking, and the subsequent secretion by these macrophages of a proteolytic enzyme which dissolves lung tissue
- recurrent infection in the lungs causing inflammation and fibrosis
- small airways obstruction
- loss of elastic recoil of lung tissue caused by tobacco smoke inhibition of alpha-antitrypsin – this enzyme is normally responsible for preventing the action of the proteolytic enzymes in the lungs breaking down the lung tissue.

The syndrome of chronic bronchitis, therefore, displays a graduation of severity:

---

hypersecretion of mucus from hypertrophic bronchial glands
↓
inflammatory changes caused by secondary infections
↓
narrowing of bronchial and bronchiolar airways
↓
emphysema
↓
pulmonary hypertension
↓
cardiac failure (cor pulmonale)

Causes

There are numerous clues in the chronic bronchitis story which, when pieced together, are beginning to show what might be possible to prevent and control in a prevalent and disabling condition.

Age and sex

It is a condition of ageing and presumably of degeneration of the respiratory tract that has been subjected to years of irritation by atmospheric pollutants, inhaled pathogenic organisms and, in smokers, to many years of self-inhaled irritants.

It is more frequent in males than in females and the mortality rates are also higher ($\times 2$ in the UK) in males. However, the excessive prevalence of chronic bronchitis in males is more apparent in those under 65, and the sex differences become less notable in the elderly.

Geography

Traditionally chronic bronchitis has been labelled as the 'English disease' and international mortality rates show that the United Kingdom apparently has the worst record for chronic bronchitis. However, when comparative international surveys are carried out, using standardized questionnaires, these mortality differences became less, because of correction of terminological differences.

It may well be that the British climate, housing and other social habits are responsible for some differences, but customs and habits of disease nomenclature and labelling are also a major reason for the difference.

Urban-rural differences: British studies have shown that there is a definite higher prevalence (2 : 1) of chronic bronchitis in urban compared with rural areas.

In this context atmospheric pollution and climate are important causal factors. The greater the pollution the higher the rates of chronic bronchitis. The most severe and acute effects on the respiratory tract came from English fogs with their dirt, cold and damp. They are now rare, benefits of Clean Air Policy.

Social class

Unexplained are the higher prevalence, morbidity, severity and mortality of chronic bronchitis in the lower social classes. In Britain the mortality from chronic bronchitis in unskilled labourers (social class V) is four times greater than in professional men (social class I), but not only is the mortality greater in the men, the same social class gradients exist also in their wives.

Smoking

Smoking has decreased by almost one-half in the adult population from over 60% in 1950s–60s to 33% now. It is higher in lower social groups and although still higher in men the rates in young women are equal to young men, around 40%.

15–20% of smokers seem particularly susceptible to the tobacco smoke with respect to the development of small airway obstruction. When a smoker with impaired lung function stops smoking, there is no recovery of the lost lung function, but the rate of subsequent further decline gradually becomes similar to those who have never smoked.

Occupation

Dusty occupations may lead to the production of excessive mucus and eventually small airway obstruction.

Genetic factors

This may lead to a deficiency of the enzyme, alpha-antitrypsin, which prevents proteolytic damage to the lungs.

Asthma

Childhood asthma may be a factor, as a past history of asthma is associated with an increased susceptibility of the lungs to tobacco smoke.

Allergy

Allergy and bronchial hypersensitivity may be contributory factors in some patients.

Who gets it and when?

The prevalence of 'chronic bronchitis' as a diagnostic label is declining. This may only be *apparent* because the diagnosis has become less popular and more are being diagnosed alternatively as asthma, emphysema and chronic obstructive airways disease (COAD). However, there may have been a *real* decline because of reduction in smoking, less atmospheric pollution and better housing and personal environmental conditions at work and at home.

The *true prevalence of chronic bronchitis* as defined (on page 96) can only be assessed through community surveys and question-naires because the majority with 'productive cough for 3 months in the year for at least 2 consecutive years' do not consult and either treat themselves or accept the condition as a minor, normal, abnormality.

It is likely that about 25% of persons over 45 in the UK have chronic bronchitis, as defined.

Since half of the population in the UK is over 45 this means that 6 million persons have chronic bronchitis! Translated to general practice:

- in a practice of 2000 patients there are likely to be over 200 chronic bronchitics but only about 50 will consult their GP in a year
- in a practice of 10 000 patients there will be 1000 chronic bronchitics and 250 will consult in a year.

Of those who do consult with chronic bronchitis:

50 per cent will have simple bronchitis (see page 100)
20 per cent will have acute infections
30 per cent will have complicated forms.

Chronic bronchitis prevalence increases with age, and at all ages it is more frequent in men.

How does it present?

There are two basic clinical symptoms – productive cough (with sputum) and breathlessness.

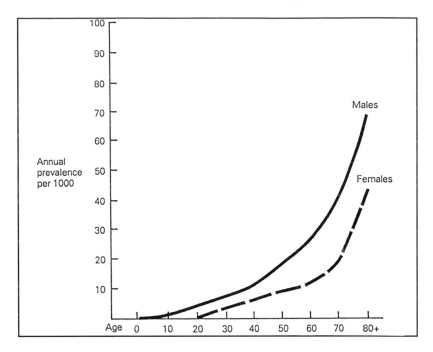

Fig. 9.1—Chronic bronchitis – prevalence

Clinically there are four *grades and categories*:

- simple chronic bronchitis
- acute on chronic bronchitis
- severe complicated disease
- respiratory failure.

Simple chronic bronchitis

Cough at first only on rising in morning with 'chest clearing' but worse in winter months and then with time cough becomes more persistent.

Sputum is mucoid but becomes readily mucopurulent with infection.

Breathlessness is variable; usually on effort and worse on cold and foggy days. Becomes progressively worse with time and occurs with normal daily functions. May waken at night. Wheezing associated with exertion, after coughing and on lying down.

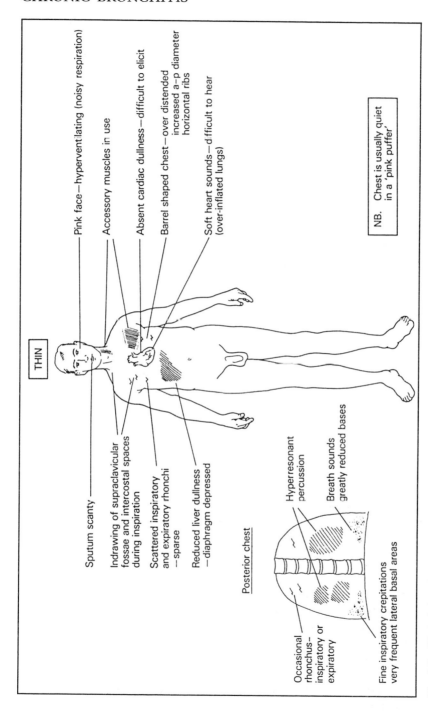

THIN

Pink face—hyperventilating (noisy respiration)

Accessory muscles in use

Absent cardiac dullness—difficult to elicit

Barrel shaped chest—over distended
increased a–p diameter
horizontal ribs

Soft heart sounds—difficult to hear
(over-inflated lungs)

NB. Chest is usually quiet
in a 'pink puffer'

Sputum scanty

Indrawing of supraclavicular
fossae and intercostal spaces
during inspiration

Scattered inspiratory
and expiratory rhonchi
—sparse

Reduced liver dullness
—diaphragm depressed

Posterior chest

Hyperresonant
percussion

Breath sounds
greatly reduced bases

Occasional
rhonchus—
inspiratory or
expiratory

Fine inspiratory crepitations
very frequent lateral basal areas

Fig. 9.2—Clinical signs in a 'pink puffer'

Acute on chronic bronchitis

Occurs with secondary infection following colds and other viral upper respiratory infections:

- increase in cough and breathlessness
- yellow-green sputum
- wheezing with generalized rhonchi and possibly local crepitations.

Severe complicated disease

Major complications are:

- severe emphysema – the *'pink puffer'* with clinical features as in Figure 9.2. These are:
  pink skin
  noisy heavy breathing
  scanty mucoid sputum
  distended chest
  elevated hunched shoulders
  accessory respiratory muscles used.
- R. ventricular failure – *the 'blue-bloater'* (Figure 9.3):
  blue and cyanosed
  quiet shallow breathing
  profuse mucopurulent sputum
  R. side cardiac failure signs
  generalized rhonchi.
- The two types may exist together.

Respiratory failure

Usually precipitated by acute infection but may be progression from the complicated types:

- increased breathlessness usual, but less so in 'blue-bloater'
- episodic bouts of sleep apnoea
- drowsiness, confusion, agitation
- headache and lack of concentration
- bounding pulse, often arrhythmias
- warm hands and feet
- hypotension and eventual circulatory collapse
- blood gases
  raised pCO_2
  lower pO_2.

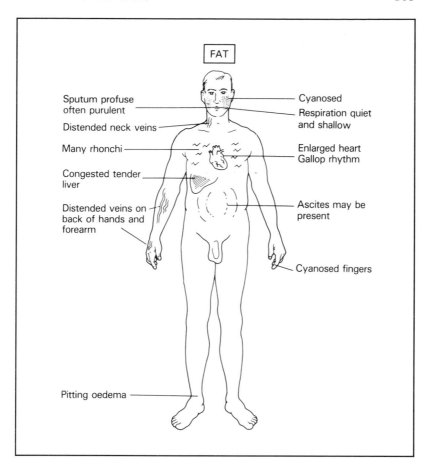

Fig. 9.3—Clinical signs in a 'blue bloater'

What happens?

There is no single pattern of natural history, but the following fits the majority of cases.

In some, a small minority (10%), the chronic bronchitis can be related back to severe and recurrent childhood chest infections. On occasions, chronic bronchitis in adults may date from a severe attack of acute bronchitis or pneumonia in a person with no previous history of chest illness. In the majority the symptoms of chronic bronchitis, persistent productive cough, begin insidiously as a smoker's cough in the patient's 40s and 50s, and once there, unless drastic measures are taken, the condition embarks on a long and chronic course for 20, 30 or 40 years.

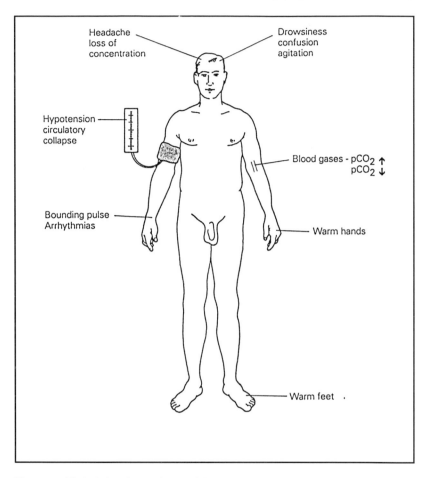

Headache loss of concentration

Drowsiness confusion agitation

Hypotension circulatory collapse

Blood gases - pCO_2 ↑
pCO_2 ↓

Bounding pulse Arrhythmias

Warm hands

Warm feet .

Fig. 9.4—Clinical signs in respiratory failure

Although more chronic bronchitics will die from chest and associated heart conditions than non-chronic bronchitics, chronic bronchitis is not a dramatic killer. It is true that 35 000 persons die from chronic bronchitis each year in the United Kingdom and three-quarters of these are over 65.

Taking the condition as a whole it is fair to state that:

• One-half of chronic bronchitics will continue to live their allotted life span with a persistent productive cough but with no appreciable functional disability.

• One-quarter will become moderately disabled with appreciable loss of respiratory function and be somewhat restricted in their

work and hobbies. They will suffer from recurrent chest infections and will be absent from work for a month or more each year.
• One-quarter will become severely disabled either quickly (only a few) or more slowly (the majority in this group) over 5–10 years.

Survival is related to the level of the forced expiratory volume at one second ($FEV_{1.0}$), e.g. a $FEV_{1.0}$ which is about 30–50% of the predicted normal, is associated with a median survival of only 5 years.

Mortality is also associated with the number of cigarettes smoked – there is a twofold difference in survival between a light smoker (<15/day) and a heavy smoker (>25/day).

Pipe and cigar smokers also show an increased mortality compared with non-smokers, but the difference is not as marked as with cigarettes.

Smoking accounts overall for about 80% of the total mortality from chronic obstructive lung disease in the affluent Western countries. If smoking stops there is no significant reduction in mortality until about 10 years later.

In a year in a practice of 2000 patients

• 200 chronic bronchitics
• 50 consult GP
• 20 will suffer acute–chronic chest infection
• 5 will be admitted to hospital
• 1 or 2 will die.

What to do?

Chronic bronchitis is common in the UK. There are many underlying causes but smoking, atmospheric pollution and occupational hazards are the most important.

It has a long course with appreciable disability and mortality for some.

There is much that the GP can do in encouraging patients not to smoke and to advise on occupational hazards and in managing the effects and complications.

Differential diagnosis

Before accepting a diagnosis of 'chronic bronchitis' it is important to consider and exclude other serious conditions with similar clinical features:

- *chronic asthma* which may merge with chronic bronchitis
- *cancer of bronchus* – similar causal factor of smoking and may affect persons with chronic bronchitis
- *pulmonary tuberculosis* – should be considered in recent immigrants from Asia and Africa and in elderly men with decline in health and cough.

Investigations

Chest X-ray

Although there are few specific features in chronic bronchitis a chest X-ray should be considered to exclude cancer and tuberculosis. Presence of emphysema can be demonstrated.

Respiratory function tests

These are important to assess the extent of functional disability and check response to treatment.

Sputum examination

This is of little practical help apart from diagnosis of pulmonary tuberculosis.

ECG

ECG is helpful in confirming diagnosis of complicating cardiac failure.

Assessment of functional state

A good guide to the state of respiratory function lies in the patient's history and his ability to carry out normal activities. Regular objective checks, however, are a useful means of recording progress or deterioration and to measure the response to treatment and preventive actions.

Two practical and simple tests of respiratory function are the Peak Flow Meter that measures the peak expiratory flow rate

(PEFR) and the Vitalograph Spirometer which will measure forced vital capacity (FVC) and forced expiratory volume (FEV) in one second.

Peak expiratory flow rate

This is related to changes in the larger central airways and is therefore not a particularly sensitive method of assessing small airway obstruction. However, it is simple and convenient and can be measured easily by the patient at home with a mini-peak flow meter, and is therefore in widespread use.

Spirometry

This is a more accurate measure of small airway obstruction, and the $FEV_{1.0}$ is the best measure of its degree. The other measurement made on the spirometer is the forced vital capacity, but it is likely that a better guide would be the 'relaxed' vital capacity, since the act of forcing the expiration can itself cause spasm and narrowing of the small airways.

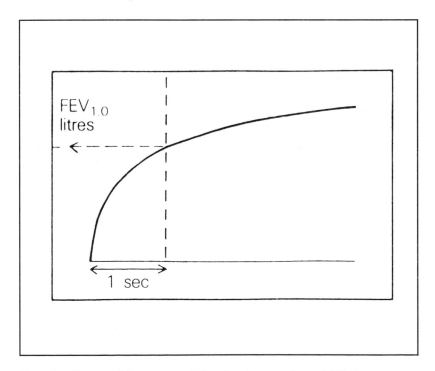

Fig. 9.5—Diagram of the one-second forced expiratory volume ($FEV_{1.0}$)

Exercise test

A 10–12 minute walking test is sometimes of value in assessing the severity of impairment of lung function in chronic bronchitis, the assessment being made on the number of stops required during the walk.

Management of chronic bronchitis

The types of treatment available for chronic bronchitis are:

- specific therapy
- prophylactic therapy
- symptomatic therapy
- additional supportive therapy.

Specific treatment

STOP SMOKING advice for the patient and his relatives:

- self-help literature
- self-help groups
- hypnosis/acupuncture helps some patients.

Look for α_1-antitrypsin deficiency, especially in young patients with chronic bronchitis, and particularly if there is a strong family history of chronic bronchitis. Although there is no specific treatment available for this as yet, some encouraging results have been obtained in the USA from infusion of the enzyme intravenously.

Prophylactic treatment

- *STOP SMOKING* – this is as important for prophylaxis as for specific treatment
- control of atmospheric pollution, especially from petrol-driven vehicles. This is currently a subject of much concern and some efforts are being made to control this factor, especially in the manufacture of these vehicles
- avoid group contacts in the flu season, and going out in inclement weather conditions, especially fogs
- avoid obesity

- vaccines:
  pneumococcal capsular polysaccharide vaccine may be useful in elderly patients to prevent pneumoccocal infection
  flu vaccine may be of value in some patients with chronic lung disease in proven-acute exacerbations (see Chapter 3)
- antibiotics – a good case can be made out for susceptible patients to have available a supply of an appropriate antibiotic to use at the first sign of a lung infection, and the best guide to this is the development of green or yellow sputum.

Symptomatic (relief) treatment

Cough and sputum: There is no known reliable way of reducing the volume of sputum. There are no good proven measures of reducing the distressing stickiness of sputum.

There are many cough mixtures and medicines, and their multitude is evidence of their lack of success. However, each physician should select some mixtures that may be given to sufferers in order to relieve some symptoms. A simple linctus and a few expectorant mixtures can be selected and used for these purposes, often in the knowledge that their action will be more as placebos than specifics.

Airway obstruction – the main bronchodilators available are:

---

(1) beta₁-sympathetic agonists
(2) anticholinergic drugs
(3) methylxanthine derivatives.

---

(1) *Beta₁-agonists*:

- Drugs such as salbutamol or terbutaline are the agonists used most frequently. In severe cases these drugs are best given by nebulizer which is now available for home use.
- The newer long-acting salmeterol may be used b.d., instead of q.d.s. as with salbutamol or at night before going to bed to prevent nocturnal wheezing.
- The delivery systems available for these drugs include:
  metered-dose inhalers, which are the most widely used, but in 30–50% of patients technique is deficient
  spacer devices – useful if there is poor coordination in the use of the metered-dose inhaler
  dry powder inhalation
  nebulizer – more efficient than the metered-dose inhaler and is now available for use at home through the NHS.

If none of these devices is usable in a patient, then the beta-agonist can be given orally, but is more likely to produce side-effects due to sympathetic over-activity.

There is no convincing evidence that beta-agonists improve the long-term prognosis in chronic obstructive airway diseases.

(2) *Ipratropium* – this is an anticholinergic drug which interferes with bronchoconstriction mediated through the vagus nerves. It is usually taken in a metered-dose inhaler but can also be used in a nebulizer. It has a slower onset of action than a beta-sympathetic agonist, from 30 to 60 minutes, but is sometimes effective where the beta-agonist fails. Side-effects include urinary retention, so care should be taken in elderly male patients with probable prostate problems.

(3) *Methylxanthines* – these drugs include theophylline and its derivatives. They act as bronchodilators and mild respiratory stimulants. Their main problem is the narrow margin between a therapeutic dose and a toxic dose, so close attention should be paid to the blood levels of the drug. They are of limited value in chronic airflow obstructions.

Steroid treatment: Steroids can be tried if there is an inadequate response to maximum bronchodilator treatment.

If steroids are used it is important to monitor the effects by a diary card and by regular measurement of the peak flow rates. The steroid can be tried initially in a metered-dose inhaler, e.g. beclomethasone, which can be tried in increasing doses, from 500–1000 mg daily, but if this fails, then a course of oral steroids is justified. Prednisolone is usually given in a dose of 30–40 mg daily for 10 to 14 days; the full dose can be given daily or the dose can be progressively tapered off over the treatment period – the benefits are the same. The effects should be carefully monitored by peak flow rates and if the improvement is less than 25%, the prednisolone should be withdrawn. Side-effects resulting from this short course are rare.

Anoxaemia: Severely breathless bronchitics are helped by having access to supplies of oxygen at home. Oxygen concentrators with the necessary masks and other equipment are prescribable and are available under the British NHS.

The long-term prognosis can be improved by administering oxygen, but it needs to be taken continuously for a minimum period of 15 hours in the day.

Another helpful use of oxygen is just before exercise to enable the effort to be made with less distress.

Rehabilitation and occupation

The problem of rehabilitation of a disabled bronchitic is a great challenge that is only rarely overcome.

Fitting a late middle-aged man into a new and protected job is far from easy, particularly during a high unemployment period.

What usually happens is that early premature retirement becomes necessary and the patient then has to be helped to busy himself with hobbies or part-time work, either at home or within a short distance of his home.

Social services and assistance: There are a number of forms of assistance and help that can be given to disabled chronic bronchitics, such as mobility allowances, supplementary benefits and attendance allowances in severe cases.

General management: Although there is no cure for established chronic bronchitis, the physician can do much to relieve and comfort his severe chronic bronchitic patients. Of first priority are measures to prevent deterioration and to improve function, by stopping smoking and avoidance of severe and inclement climatic conditions. The bronchitics should not tempt fate by going out in cold and damp foggy weather. An even and warm temperature should be achieved in their homes during the winter months. Regular support by the physician by regular contact either at the consulting room or through home visiting of housebound respiratory invalids is important and appreciated. Such regular visits can be shared between the physician and his nurse and social worker. This support is needed not only by the patient but also by his family.

Reduction of obesity – obesity increases respiratory demands and reduces respiratory efficiency.

A *program of physical training* may be of psychological value, and activity should be encouraged as far as possible.

Summary of treatment of an acute exacerbation of chronic bronchitis

- Intensive bronchodilator therapy by metered-dose inhaler or nebulizer if necessary.
- Start antibiotics and assess response on the colour of the sputum.
- Course of oral steroids if no improvement with maximum bronchodilator therapy.
- Physiotherapy to help get rid of retained secretions.

Cor pulmonale

Clinical definition

Although the World Health Organization defines cor pulmonale as right ventricular hypertrophy associated with chronic lung disease, in practice it is taken to mean right ventricular failure due to chronic lung disease.

It occurs in about 10% of patients with severe chronic obstructive lung disease, and is associated with a very poor prognosis – most patients die within 2 years.

Clinical findings

The typical signs are those of the 'blue bloater' (see pages 103). These patients usually manifest also some signs of respiratory failure:

- depressed respiration
- drowsiness and sometimes confusion
- headache
- peripheral vasodilatation with a bounding pulse and poor blood pressure;
- flapping tremor
- fundi – venous engorgement, sometimes papilloedema.

The most important test for diagnosing respiratory failure is the arterial level of the pCO$_2$ which is above 6 kPa.

Management of cor pulmonale and respiratory failure

- Consider admission to hospital
- Antibiotic – usually amoxycillin to start
- Diuretic – frusemide 40 mg i.v. initially. Can add spironolactone and/or an ACE inhibitor. Metolazone can also be added if the frusemide is ineffective – it is a powerful thiazide which can greatly enhance the diuretic effect of the frusemide
- Bronchodilator therapy – best by nebulizer
- Steroid treatment – parenteral and/or oral
- Controlled oxygen
- Physiotherapy
- Positive pressure ventilation if deterioration continues and this is best assessed by measuring the blood gases

Practical points

- Chronic bronchitis is defined as productive cough with daily sputum for 3 months for at least 2 consecutive years.
- By this definition one-quarter of over-45s in the UK have chronic bronchitis.
- Diagnosis is imprecise and there is a need to exclude cancer of bronchus and pulmonary tuberculosis with similar features.
- Four grades: simple bronchitis, acute on chronic, severe complicated and respiratory failure.
- Major causes are smoking, atmospheric pollution and occupational hazards – so it should be preventable.
- One-half of simple chronic bronchitics live normal life spans, one-quarter become moderately disabled and one-quarter seriously disabled.
- In a practice of 2000 patients there are 200 chronic bronchitics but only 50 will consult each year, 5 will be admitted to hospital and 1 or 2 die.
- Prevention is the target with cessation of smoking most important.
- Chest X-ray for exclusion of other serious diseases and peak flow for assessment of function and grade are most useful in investigations.
- Apart from prevention, treatment is towards relief with antispasmodics, steroids and oxygen and treatment of complications such as infections, cardiac and respiratory failure.

CHAPTER **10**

ASTHMA

What is it?

Although we have a vague understanding of what 'asthma' is, when this understanding becomes subjected to more careful analysis, difficulties of definition soon appear. A common definition of asthma is that it is a state of recurrent and paroxysmal bouts of chest wheezing and breathlessness, and characterized by wide variations in resistance to airflow in the bronchial airway for short periods of time. This is quite accurate but there are a number of syndromes that can be separated from within such a definition. The truism that 'all that wheezes is not asthma' is apt.

These *acute wheezy chests* (AWC) comprise the following groups:

(1) Acute wheezy chests in young children (see page 53). These attacks of wheezing and breathlessness are part of the 'catarrhal child syndrome' and are associated with a triggering infection. About one-quarter of all children suffer acute wheezy chests, but only 10% of these go on to 'asthma' after the age of 15.
(2) Acute exacerbations in chronic bronchitis (see page 102). Bouts of wheezing and breathlessness in chronic bronchitis are not infrequent and whilst some are associated with infection, others are part of the progression of the chronic bronchitic condition. It is probable that about one-quarter of chronic bronchitics will suffer these acute bouts.

114

(3) Rarely, a localized obstruction of a bronchus may cause bouts of wheezing and breathlessness. Such a situation may result from a growing cancer of the bronchus that may for a time cause intermittent bronchial obstruction: an inhaled foreign body may produce similar effects and swelling of hilar lymph glands may also produce similar symptoms and signs.

(4) Finally, almost by a process of exclusion, we arrive at the condition of asthma, but there are difficulties in deciding which wheezy children are potential future asthmatics and whether some chronic bronchitic wheezers are the result of long-standing asthma.

Asthma can be viewed as an individual 'diathesis' or make-up with a hyper-reactive respiratory tract and many possible 'triggers' and factors.

It is customary to subdivide asthma into atopic (intrinsic) and non-atopic (extrinsic) types.

- *Atopic asthma* has an early onset with episodic attacks and often a family history of allergic disorders. The children are likely also to suffer from eczema.
- *Non-atopic asthma* has a late (adult) onset, persistent breathlessness with severe acute attacks and no family history.

The associated aetiological factors include:

- family history in 25% of atopic asthmatics
- hay fever in 30% (7% in non-asthmatics)
- vasomotor rhinitis in 20% (5% in non-asthmatics)
- childhood eczema in 15% of atopics (5% in non-asthmatics)
- history of anxiety, depression and stress in 40% (12% in non-asthmatics)
- history of maternal smoking before and after birth
- lower maternal age
- large families
- specific allergens include house dust mite, animal hair or feathers, pollens, moulds, foods and occupational exposure to metal salts, drugs and vegetable dusts.

Whatever the causal factors, the pathological changes involve spasm and constriction of bronchioles, excessive secretion of bronchial thick and sticky mucus and mucosal swelling and oedema.

Who gets it and when?

For the whole population the age prevalence shows that asthma is most frequent in the young and the elderly. A practice with 2000 persons can expect in a year:

- 2 new cases of asthma
- 40 persons with asthma (with 60–80 attacks)
- 200 potential asthmatics with present or past history.

Children

The age prevalence in the first 10 years shows high rates in early childhood and school years with some decline after the age of seven. Up to 25% of children suffer one or more bouts of chest-wheezing, usually part of an acute respiratory infection. Of these:

- 70% have minor episodes not requiring treatment;
- 25% have significant attacks needing medical advice;
- 5% have troublesome asthma requiring continuing therapy.

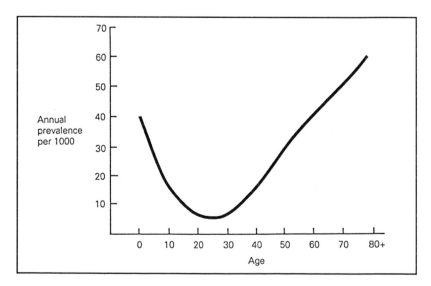

Fig. 10.1—Asthma – age prevalence of all acute wheezy chests

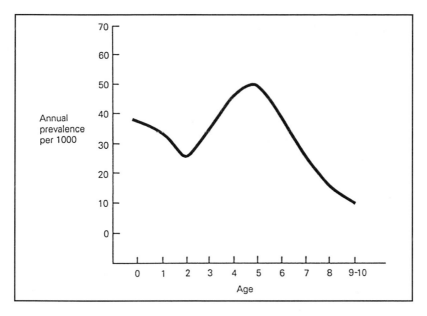

Fig. 10.2—Asthma – age prevalence of acute wheezy chests in children (0–10 years)

Adults

The annual consulting rate for asthma in adults is 15 per 1000 with peaks in early adult life and after 60 (Figure 10.4).

In the *elderly* there is a close relationship to 'chronic bronchitis' and rates increase with age (Figure 10.5).

The diagnosis of 'asthma' has become more popular among doctors and more acceptable to patients. This may account for the increase in prevalence rates. However, this increase may be real resulting from new and greater causal factors possibly atmospheric pollution and allergens.

How does it present?

Prominent features are:

- persistent cough in children that is worse at night
- episodic attacks of chest tightness, breathlessness, wheezing and cough with sticky sputum
- variation of symptoms, often worse in early hours or on waking.

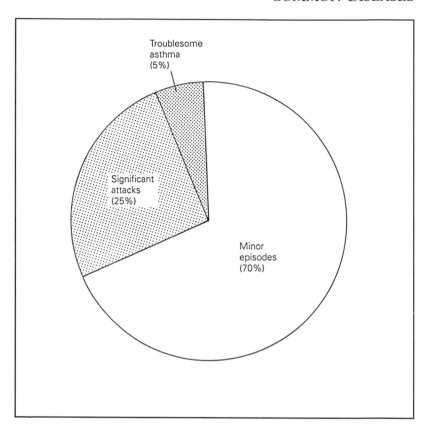

Figure 10.3—Bouts of chest-wheezing in children – grades of severity

Attacks may be spontaneous but are often brought on by triggers such as colds and flu-like illnesses, allergens (see page 115), cold air, smoke and fumes, aerosols, exercise (in children and young adults), drugs such as salicylates, NSAIDs and beta-blockers and foods with tartrazine dyes.

Severity ranges from a minor nuisance to a life-threatening situation:

- *Minor attacks* – persistent cough, wheezing and breathlessness.
- *Moderate attack* – marked breathlessness, use of accessory muscles of respiration, hyper-resonant chest and generalized high pitched wheezes.
- *Severe* – extreme breathlessness, cannot lie down, holding chair or bed to fix shoulder girdle for support, unable to talk, pale and sweating, weak rapid pulse.

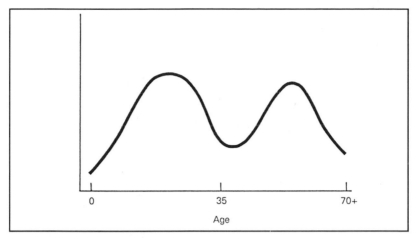

Fig. 10.4—Asthma (adult onset) – two peaks of prevalence, in early adult life and in late life

Particular danger signs are confusion and drowsiness, cyanosis, silent chest and slowing pulse.

Note: if the peak expiratory flow rate is 50% below patient's usual readings and fails to improve with bronchodilators then urgent hospitalization is imperative.

What happens?

The natural history of asthma is best recorded under the three clinical types:

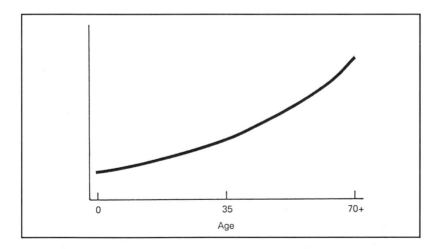

Fig. 10.5—Chronic bronchitic 'wheezers' rise with age

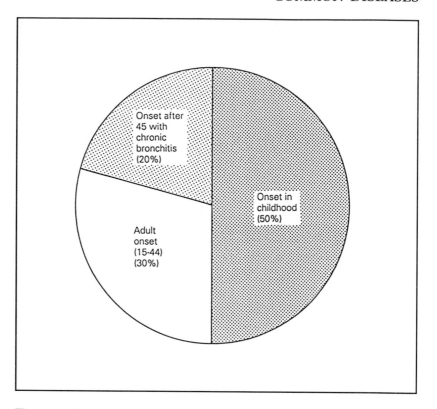

Fig. 10.6—The three clinical types of asthma

- early onset in childhood (50% of all asthma)
- adult onset at ages 15–44 (30%)
- late onset associated with chronic bronchitis after 45 (20%).

Childhood onset asthma

As noted (page 53), about 1 in 4 children suffer at least one acute wheezy chest. Of these, 80% start before the age of 7. The outcome is:

- 50% no attacks by adolescence
- 33% are prone to occasional minor attacks
- 15% have frequent attacks
- 2% are disabled requiring constant therapy with some loss of pulmonary function.

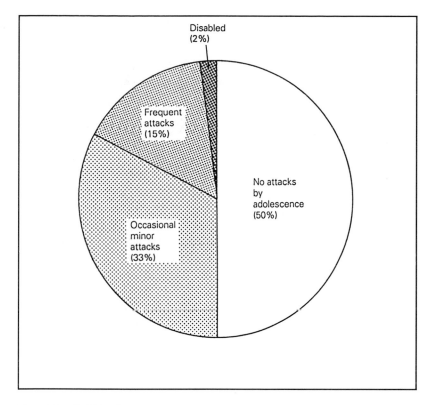

Fig. 10.7—Childhood onset asthma – outcome

The outcomes are related to the severity of asthma in childhood. Four-fifths of severe childhood asthmatics continue into adult life but only one-fifth of those with mild asthma continue.

Adult onset asthma

The outcome in late onset asthma is less good:

- 30% cease to suffer attacks after 10–15 years
- 30% continue with occasional minor attacks
- 30% have frequent attacks with some functional disability
- 10% become respiratory invalids on constant treatment and with appreciable decline in function.

Chronic bronchitics

The outlook is poor.
Once wheezing has occurred then:
- 75% will suffer attacks annually with some functional disability
- 25% will become severely and progressively disabled.

Prognostic factors

- *Smoking* is a major aggravating factor in outcome. This may be smoking by the asthmatic or by the parents of asthmatic children (passive smoking).
- *Severity of the condition* – the more frequent and the more severe the attacks the more likely a *poor outlook*.
- *Atopic children* with other allergies are more likely to continue attacks into adult life than non-atopics.
- *Family history* of asthma, allergies or chronic chest disease makes for a less good prognosis.
- *Treatment* – it is unclear whether long-term and continuing treatment with powerful drugs such as steroids or beta-agonists makes for a better or worse outcome.
- *Seasonal*: autumn and winter months are times for more severe attacks (apart from those with summer allergies such as hay fever) because of fall in ambient temperature, increase in house dust mites, autumnal fungus spores and more respiratory cross-infections.

Mortality

With 40 asthmatics consulting a GP with 2000 patients annually this means approximately 1.3 million in the UK.

For the past decade there have been around 2200 deaths from asthma each year. This represents an annual mortality rate of 1 per 590 consulting asthmatics. However most deaths (2000) occur in the more severe and chronic asthmatics (about 200 000 in the UK) and in these the annual mortality rate is 1 per 100 With 33 000 GPs this implies about one death from asthma every 15 years.

In theory all these deaths should be preventable but many occur unexpectedly in asthmatics already under long-term care.

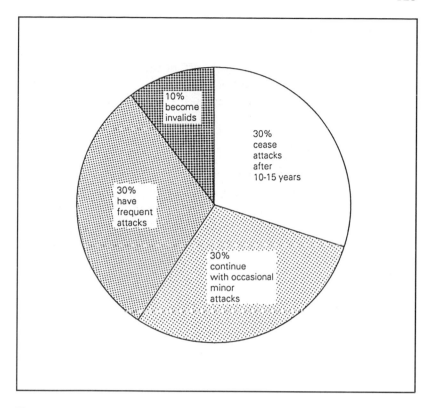

Fig. 10.8—Adult onset asthma – outcome

What to do?

Assessment

In an assessment of an asthmatic patient the following points should be considered
(1) What type of individual is he and what family background does he have?
(2) What type of asthma is he suffering from? Is he in fact suffering from asthma?
(3) Are there any definable causes or triggers?
(4) Are any such causes or triggers preventable?

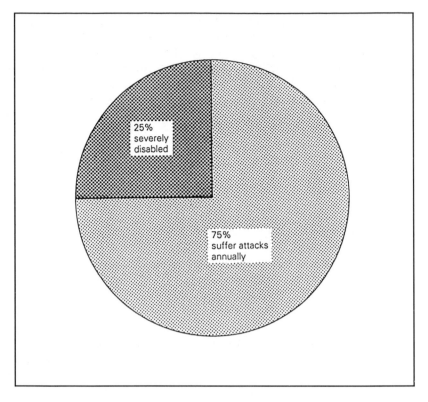

Fig. 10.9—Chronic bronchitis – outlook

(5) What is the functional state and how might it be improved?

- wheezing every week
- wheezing at night every week
- interference with lifestyle.

(6) What programme of management should be organized?

The personal and family characteristics are helpful in assessment and management. Asthmatics tend to be more anxious and nervous than average. Whether this is the result of recurrent asthmatic attacks or a basic constitutional feature is not certain. It is a fact that asthmatics more than other patients require continuing personal care from a physician in whom they have confidence, and it is important that such a personal doctor–patient relationship be built up for sound care that probably will extend over many years.

Diagnosis of asthma must be accurate, particularly in late-onset adult asthma, and other causes of wheezing such as cancer of the lung, fibrosing alveolitis, left-sided cardiac failure and chronic bronchitis and emphysema, should be excluded by chest radiography and, if necessary, by further investigations.

Prognostically, determination of the type of asthma is useful in assessing the type of management required.

Early-onset asthma is characterized by onset in childhood and a family and personal history of associated allergies such as hay fever and eczema. The respiratory functional state is good between attacks and the outcome usually is excellent. Very few, only 1 in 50, become severely disabled.

Later-onset asthma begins in middle age. There is usually no personal or family history of associated allergies. There is a merging association with chronic bronchitis, and often it is difficult to discover which came first, the chronic bronchitis or the asthma. The outcome is much worse than in the early-onset asthma. More than 1 in 10 will experience progressive deterioration of respiratory function and invalidism.

Wherever possible causal triggers should be detected in order to be avoided. This is not easy. Good history and recording of associated circumstances of each attack by the patient and family are more likely to reveal such factors than more sophisticated tests for allergens, such as skin tests and challenge of inhaled allergens.

If causes can be defined then avoidance should be attempted. This may prove difficult. Dust should be reduced to a minimum and possible bed mites and their eggs may be avoided by plastic covering of mattresses and pillows. Contact with sensitizing animals may be avoided also. The value of specific desensitizing courses by injection with increasing doses of allergens may work dramatically in a few instances but in the majority the results are not worth the risks, discomforts and extra work.

Good management of asthmatics requires regular *measurements and recording* of *respiratory function* and a *plan* of *management* that should be understood and followed by patients and relatives.

In some asthmatics attacks may be *prevented* by avoiding known causes or by using appropriate medication, such as a bronchodilator aerosol before exercise; attacks may be *aborted* by effective and early treatment in which the asthmatic has been instructed; more severe cases require *continuing treatment* with trials of various therapies; a few are so severely disabled and housebound that help with *continuous oxygen* is necessary.

Investigations

Respiratory function tests

The most important investigation is the respiratory function test involving the use of either a Vitalograph in hospital for a more detailed assessment, or the peak expiratory flow mini-meter which can be used by the patient in his home. This test can be used in children from 7–8 years of age but is unreliable below this age.

The important measurements in this test are the peak expiratory flow rate (PEFR) and the forced expiratory volume at one second ($FEV_{1.0}$) – either should show at least 20% improvement with an inhaled bronchodilator to confirm a diagnosis of asthma. The other important benefit of this test is in showing the response to treatment.

Chest X-ray is usually normal in asthma and is not indicated as a routine. It may be appropriate when a differential diagnosis is being considered or when a complication such as pneumonia is suspected during acute attacks in adults with more than expected breathlessness.

Skin tests for allergy; *blood tests* for eosinophilia and raised IgE, or *provocation tests* with histamine or methacholine are all unhelpful in normal practice.

Management

Asthma is a condition that, once started, will go on for some years before, hopefully, improving naturally. Therefore, once diagnosed it is essential that plans and preparations are made for the long-term care of the patient and his family

Conditions such as asthma are managed most easily if there are good relations between physician and patient and where there is a good understanding of the nature and course and probable outcome by both patient and physician.

Once diagnosed it is important that time be spent in 'educating and informing' the patient and relatives in simple terms of the situation, the course and the aims of treatment, emphasizing the good likely prognosis and the need to lead as normal a life as possible in spite of the inconvenient acute episodes of asthma.

The aims of the personal physician must be to develop self-confidence and prevent fears and anxieties in his asthmatic patients, and to teach them how to manage the acute attacks that unfortunately will occur at times.

Although asthmatics do become anxious and depressed, probably as a result of the stresses of the illness rather than because of some defective make-up, it should not be necessary to treat these anxieties and depressions with long-term tranquilizers or antidepressants. Good personal care, understanding and support are more effective than psychotropic pills.

General measures

- Educate patient/relative in:
  nature of asthma
  possible causes/triggers
  what treatment can/cannot do
  correct use of peak flow meter
  when to summon medical help
  how to manage treatment themselves, especially with the use of the peak flow meter.
- Counselling for emotional problems.
- Anti-allergic treatment – only of value if the allergen is known. Other non-specific measures such as room cleaning, special bedclothes, removal of domestic animals is unlikely to be of much benefit.
- Desensitization – no long-term benefits have been shown, and significant morbidity, and occasional deaths, have occurred from the injection of the allergen.
- Exercise programmes – swimming is widely recommended as unlikely to cause exercise-induced asthma, probably because of the warm, moist environment. It may be of psychological value to the patient.

Specific treatment – drug therapy

Drugs used:

- *Beta$_2$-agonists* – mainstay of treatment in most patients with asthma, they are relatively safe and all equally effective, eg. salbutamol, terbutaline.
- *Sodium cromoglycate* – effective prophylactic especially when an allergic basis in suspected – also useful in preventing exercise-induced asthma.
- *Steroids* – inhaled steroids are the mainstay of treatment in severe persisting asthma. Oral steroids are indicated in persisting acute episodic asthma, and are also occasionally necessary long-term in severe chronic asthma.

- *Theophyllines* – there is a narrow margin between therapeutic and toxic doses so careful attention to blood levels is important. Main value preventing nocturnal asthma.
- *Ipratropium* – anticholinergic drug – main benefit is in treating severe acute attacks not responding to other treatment; used in nebulizer form in these patients.
- *Antibiotics* – tend to be over-prescribed in asthma, especially in children, since there is little evidence that bacterial infection precipitates attacks. The green sputum sometimes seen in asthmatic attacks may be due to excessive eosinophils in the sputum and not indicative of bacterial infection. There is also little evidence that secondary bacterial infection is common in asthma.
- *Others* – e.g. antihistamines, cough suppressants, expectorants: there is little evidence of objective benefit in asthma but they may be of psychological help to the patient.

Treatment of a mild attack of asthma

Beta$_2$-agonist is the first line of treatment – this can be used in a metered dose inhaler as necessary. If a child – or an adult for that matter – is unable to use a metered aerosol then other options are available, such as a spacer device or a dry powder inhaler. If inhalation is not possible at all, then an oral sustained-release bronchodilator or oral slow-release theophylline can be tried

Treatment of a moderate attack of asthma

Recognized by continuation of symptoms in spite of 2–4 inhalations a day of a beta$_2$-agonist.

Inhaled bronchodilators are continual and sodium cromoglycate inhalations are added, 4-hourly.

Treatment of a severe attack of asthma

Recognized by:

- failure to respond to inhaled beta-agonists and inhaled steroids;
- tachycardia > 110/min
- difficulty in completing a sentence
- peak expiratory flow < 120 litres/min.

The patient should be *admitted urgently to hospital* for treatment with parenteral steroids, nebulizers, oxygen and fluid and electrolyte replacement.

Long-term management

To repeat - a *plan* of management should be understood and probably a *protocol* agreed by the practice team.

For the *episodic asthmatic*: appropriate use of a bronchodilator aerosol (for adults) or spacer (for children).

Note: Some asthmatics may overuse aerosols and become habituated because of anxiety over possible attacks. Frequent requests for repeat prescriptions for aerosols should be a warning signal for extra support and counselling.

For frequent and persistent asthma – a stepladder programme:

- *Bronchodilator* used regularly, the frequency determined individually:
    aerosol (or powder) for adults
    spacer for children (solution)
    nebulizer if above methods are difficult or impossible.
- *Nebulizer* can be used long-term or for acute attacks with care and supervision. Good instruction is necessary at the start and should be used in conjunction with a peak flow meter to demonstrate response.
- Oral *theophylline* may be useful for nocturnal asthma in children and adults. Single dose at bedtime.
- *Sodium cromoglycate* on a regular basis can be very effective in children and some adults with an allergic diathesis.
- If poor response to above drugs then *steroids* are indicated.
  Indications are 'all day tightness', nocturnal attacks, low quality of life and persistent low PFR readings.
  Inhaled preparation for long-term use, such as beclomethasone – which is available in measured dosage from 50 mg to 400 mg. The frequency, dosage and preparation must be adapted individually. They may be used by aerosol, powder or nebulizer.
  Oral steroids (predinsolone) or *intravenous steroids* in an emergency must be available for saving lives as well as for the occasional severe asthmatic who does not respond to other therapy.
  Oral prednisolone if no response to high doses of inhaled steroids – use lowest effective dosage and endeavour to withdraw periodically.
  Intravenous hydrocortisone should be available in 100–200 mg doses before admission to hospital in severe attacks.

Practical points

- 'Asthma' is a collection of different types of respiratory disorders with the common features of recurrent, paroxysmal or persistent chest wheezing and breathlessness and evidence of bronchial airways restriction.
- A practice of 2000 can expect two new cases each year, 40 asthmatics consult and there are 200 past and present potential cases.
- Three clinical types:
  childhood 'acute wheezy chests' – atopic and non-atopic varieties
  later onset adult asthma
  part of the chronic bronchitis syndrome.
- Outcomes vary:
  Childhood asthma – 50% have no attacks after adolescence; 33% have occasional mild attacks; 15% have frequent attacks and 2% become chronic with considerable disability.
  Adult onset – 30% cease attacks after 10–15 years, 30% have occasional minor attacks; 30% have frequent attacks; 10% chronic disability.
  Chronic bronchitics: 75% suffer annual attacks and 25% are disabled.
- *Annual mortality* of around 2200, with no fall in past 10 years. This means an annual risk of 1 in 1000 for all asthmatics but 1 in 100 for severe cases. It also means a death from asthma once every 10–12 years per GP.
- It should be possible to relieve all asthmatics with modern step by step management with:
  bronchodilators
  theophylline
  cromoglycate
  steroids
- Basis of good management is education for self-care of the asthmatic and a clear practice protocol.

CHAPTER 11

HAY FEVER AND RHINITIS

What is it?

The nose has several important physiological functions. Its sensitive nerve endings pick up and translate smells. Its convoluted mucus membrane acts as a protective filter and moisturizer of inhaled air. These actions are carried out through complex immunological reactions involving production of mucus and responses of specialized T and B lymphocytes.

With such an intricate front line defensive mechanism it is not surprising that hyper-reactions can occur, triggered by various known and unknown agents.

Just as in asthma (Chapter 10) hyper-reactivity occurs in the lower respiratory tract, so it does in the nose, the upper respiratory tract.

There are three broad common clinical conditions associated with this state of hypersensitivity:

- *hay fever* (seasonal rhinitis) where the causal allergens are specific grass, tree, shrub, weed or flower pollens or moulds
- *other specific nasal allergies* from inhaled dust, house mites and animal furs or from allergic reactions to certain foods or drugs, e.g. aspirin in some individuals

- *perennial (all year round)* rhinitis (or vasomotor rhinitis) with persistent, almost constant, symptoms of unknown cause (idiopathic).

Who gets it and when?

It is likely that some 1 in 10 of the population has some form of symptomatic allergic rhinitis.

Although this means as many as 200 persons in a practice population of 2000, not all consider it necessary to consult their doctor in any year.

The annual patient consulting rates for a practice of 2000 will be :

• hay fever	40
• other specific rhinitis	10
• perennial rhinitis	10

Hay fever has a characteristic *seasonal* occurrence from May to August in the UK. Other specific nasal allergies occur when in contact with a trigger and the perennial type is constant.

Age of onset

Hay fever: first symptoms occur in one-half of cases in the first decade and in 90% by the age of 30. Rarely it can start over the age of 60 (Figure 11.1).

Note: adult immigrants to the UK from the Caribbean, Asia and Africa commence their symptoms within 5 years of arrival.

Other specific nasal allergies have a later onset, in teens and early adult life.

Perennial rhinitis is a condition of adult life, most often commencing at ages 20–40.

How does it present?

Although the main symptoms are nasal, in *hay fever* and *other specific nasal allergies* the eyes and chest also may be affected.

Nasal: sneezing, nasal obstruction and irritation, and profuse nasal discharge.

Eyes: irritation, redness, lacrimation and photophobia.

Chest: wheezing and breathlessness when pollen counts are very high in about one-third of hay fever victims.

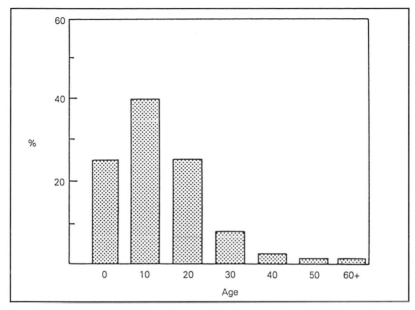

Fig. 11.1—Hay fever – age of onset

General state of misery: occurs in severe hay fever because of symptoms and also loss of sleep. All these symptoms coming together at a critical time for schoolchildren and university students can cause problems during the summer examinations.

Perennial (vasomotor) rhinitis has less dramatic, albeit distressing symptoms. The chief problems are nasal obstruction and discharge with thick sticky mucus.

Associated disorders

- *Nasal polyps* are common in persons with perennial (vasomotor) rhinitis.
- *Asthma* seasonal and inter-seasonal occurs in one third.
- *Eczema*, past or present, history in one-quarter.
- *Urticaria* in 5%.

Family history: in 20% of nasal allergic subjects there is a family history of similar or other allergies.

What happens?

All nasal allergies tend to become less troublesome and cease eventually, probably because with time the nasal mucosa loses its state of hyper-reactivity (Figure 11.2).

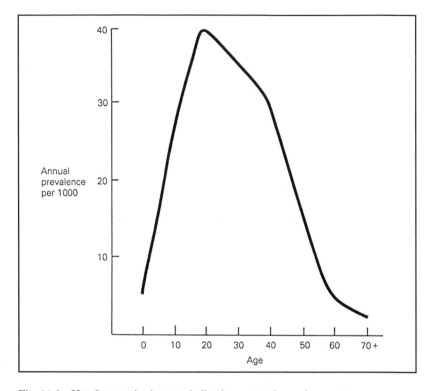

Fig. 11.2—Hay fever and other nasal allergies – annual prevalence rates

Hay fever: once started annual attacks of variable severity recur for 10–15 years and then become less troublesome and eventually cease.

Other specific rhinitis: also tends to become less troublesome after some years, probably because of decline in hyper-reactivity or because of avoidance measures.

Perennial (vasomotor) rhinitis: is likely to persist during adult life remitting after the age of 60–65. *Note*: nasal polyps occur in about 1 in 4.

What to do?

Diagnosis depends on a good *history* and assessment of symptoms relating to any possible causal triggers.

Clinical examination is not very helpful to differentiate types and causes.

Skin tests for possible allergens are of no practical value unless desensitization is being considered as a treatment.

General advice

It is important to explain the nature of the conditions and possible causes and if these can be pin-pointed then avoiding measures should be attempted – of course this is difficult with hay fever when grass pollen distribution is universal. It is also important to emphasize the natural history towards improvement and cessation of symptoms in time.

Therapeutic measures

There are no absolutely effective remedies and whilst hay fever and associated disorders do not kill, deaths have occurred from some of the treatments, such as desensitization injections and systemic steroids which can produce complications. Therefore, by all means endeavour to relieve and comfort but beware of attempts at 'cure' with potentially dangerous measures.

There are a number of popular therapeutic measures which help some individuals more than others:

- Local *nasal vasoconstrictor* nasal drops or sprays do provide temporary relief.
- *Antihistamines* – there are many oral preparations and also some for local application. They are popular but by no means universally effective and some may have unpleasant side-effects.
- *Cromoglycate* by local inhalation may help respiratory wheezing as well as nasal symptoms and also relieve eye irritation.
- *Steroids* are probably the most effective used by nasal application or inhalation by aerosol or nebulizer for wheezing, or as eye drops. With severe symptoms and faced with educational examinations and other important events it is justifiable to consider a short course of oral steroids in adequate dosage.
- *Bronchodilator aerosols* may be indicated for wheezing as in asthma (see Chapter 10).
- *Desensitization* by injections with prepared pollen is less popular because of the occasional severe allergic reactions and even death in hypersensitive subjects. If it is considered then skin tests to decide on the appropriate preparation are necessary.
- *Surgery* may be considered in severe cases of perennial (vasomotor) rhinitis including removal of nasal polyps, correction of deviated nasal septum or sub-mucous diathermy of nasal mucosa.

Practical points

- Hay fever, other forms of allergic rhinitis and perennial (vasomotor) rhinitis affect 10% of the population.
- In a year 60 patients in a practice of 2000 will consult.
- Most prevalent between 15 and 45 years of age – uncommon after 65.
- Natural course towards improvement after 10–15 years.
- No completely effective treatment.
- Popular measures include anti-histaminics, cromoglycate and steroids. Desensitization is not recommended in a general practice setting because of possible hypersensitive reactions and even death.

CHAPTER 12

CANCER OF THE LUNG

What is it?

Cancer of the lung merits a separate chapter for various reasons. It is the most frequent type of cancer in men, and second in women (after breast cancer). It causes one-quarter of all cancer deaths (40 000) each year. Five-year survival rates are less than 10%.

It poses challenges for the primary health care team:

- prevention – to stop or reduce smoking
- early diagnosis so that curative treatment may have a chance
- management that includes early referral for specialist treatment long-term personal support, terminal care.

There are *four types of lung cancer* by cell presentation and each has a different clinical picture and course:

- *Squamous cell* (epidermoid) – affects major bronchi leading to obstruction. Can cavitate and mimic lung abscess. Commonest in smokers.
- *Small (oat cell)* – rapidly invades blood vessels and lymph nodes (hilar and mediastinal). Often widely disseminated by the time the first symptoms appear.
- *Adenocarcinoma* – affects the periphery of the lung and may grow to a large size before becoming symptomatic. It may be found on routine X-ray.

- *Large cell* – consists of undifferentiated cells; locally invasive and widely disseminated.

The clinical effects of lung cancer also depend on the site, size and spread of the growth.

Locally there may be no clinical symptoms if the tumour is sited within the lung substance and does not affect the larger bronchi interfering with drainage and aeration of the distal lung tissues, or invade the lung periphery or spread to mediastinal glands which may interfere with vital structures.

Blockage of bronchi may lead to infection in the distal lung tissues or collapse and interference with ventilation and circulation through the affected lung substance.

Spread to periphery will cause invasion of the pleura or even ribs. Locally the pericardium may be involved.

Remote effects will result from metastatic spread to any part of the body. The commonest sites are mediastinal and supraclavicular lymph glands. The liver, skeleton, brain and skin are other common sites.

Systemic effects may be evident in the central nervous system, as neuropathic and myopathic syndromes. Endocrine and metabolic complications are comparatively rare and usually occur late in the course of the disease, but they may be the first signs. They result from hormones produced by the tumours. Examples are Cushing's syndrome from bilateral adrenocortical hyperplasia; hypercalcaemia from parathyroid-like hormone; hyponatraemia from secretion of antidiuretic hormone; carcinoid syndrome; hyperthyriodism; and gynaecomastia.

Hypertrophic osteoarthropathy with gross clubbing and painful fingers, feet, ankles and wrists may be an early feature.

The wide variety of possible early manifestations poses considerable tests of clinical astuteness and awareness.

Causes

There is no single cause. There is interaction between a number of causal factors. The most important proven cause is tobacco smoking, particularly cigarettes. The reasons for the different mortality rates in men and women probably are due to their different smoking rates. It is only in the past 20 years that women have been smoking as heavily as men. It seems that the latent period for development of lung cancer from heavy smoking (over 20 cigarettes per day) is over 20 years and this explains the recent progressive increase in mortality rates in women smokers.

Other causes of chronic irritation of the bronchial lining are atmospheric pollution and various industrial processes.

Smoking

There is clear evidence that the increase in lung cancer has been due to an increase in cigarette smoking – the association is with the duration of smoking and the number smoked.

In the last 10 years male smokers per total adult population have decreased from 65% to 35%, but there has been no change in the number of women smokers who remain at about 36% of the adult female population.

25% of children under 15 years old in state schools are smokers.

A higher proportion of smokers in the UK develop lung cancer than those in the USA; this is thought to be due to:

- smoking more non-filter cigarettes in the UK
- smoking down to the butt more often
- possibly associated with urban pollution.

Relevant factors in the association of smoking with lung cancer:

- Increasing incidence in women reflects the persistence of smoking in women.
- Lung cancer does occur also in non-smokers, but much less frequently.
- If a smoker of less than 20 a day stops smoking, the incidence of lung cancer declines and reaches that in non-smokers after about 13 years. When smokers of more than 20 per day stop, there is a permanent small increase in incidence of lung cancer over non-smokers.
- In smokers the predominant cancer is squamous cell; in non-smokers the predominant cancer is adenocarcinoma.
- Passive smoking may double the risk of lung cancer (300 – 400 new cases per year in USA).

Occupational factors

- radioactive materials
- asbestos★
- nickel, cadmium workers
- coal gas workers
- metallic iron and iron oxides

★Smoking cigarettes increases the risk of lung cancer fortyfold in asbestos workers.

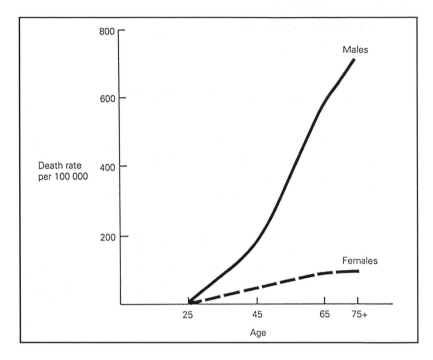

Fig. 12.1—Cancer of the lung – mortality rates

Urban pollution – probably an aetiological factor, but firm evidence lacking so far.

Who gets it and when?

Cancer of the lung occurs in adults, and its incidence increases with age.

Each year there are over 40 000 deaths in the UK (Figure 12.1) from cancer of the lung – this means 1 or 2 cases in a general practice of 2000. Since the mortality rates are 90% over 5 years, there will be the same number of *new* cases diagnosed in the practice.

At present the numbers of lung cancers are almost three times as high in men than in women, but the numbers in men are declining and numbers increasing in women, reflecting changes in smoking habits.

Britain has one of the highest rates of lung cancer in the world, probably because of smoking plus atmospheric pollution.

How does it present?

General clinical points

There are no specific symptoms of lung cancer. The clinical features depend on local, remote and systemic effects.

Local effects

Any person over 40 with persistent cough must be considered as a possible case. Chest pain, coughing up blood, breathlessness and recurring chest infections over a short period with slow resolution are even stronger reasons for urgent investigations.

Remote effects

Cancer of the lung may present or develop clinical features from metastatic spread. There may be pathological fractures; severe backache from collapse of vertebrae; headache, dementia or neurological lesions from intracranial metastases; swelling of neck from secondary gland metastases or obstruction of the superior vena cava; and skin swellings and nodules from secondary deposits.

Systemic effects

In 10–15% the first clinical features of lung cancer may be quite unrelated to the chest.

There may be general malaise, depression and loss of weight. A confusing and non-characteristic neurological picture with cerebellar or cortical disturbance, a peripheral neuropathy, myopathy or a myasthenia may be the presentation.

Unusual endocrine syndromes also may be confusing, such as complications of hypercalcaemia, carcinoid syndrome, adrenocortical hyperplasia and gynaecomastia.

Newly apparent clubbing of the fingers is now most likely to be an early feature of lung cancer, and this should be the diagnosis unless proved otherwise.

More specific clinical points

Local (primary) features

- *Cough* occurs in 80%:
  often associated with a flu-like illness or pneumonia distal to the lesion
  failure of the cough to subside is the commonest presentation.
- *Haemoptysis* occurs in 70% – should always be thoroughly investigated, especially in a smoker of 20 + cigarettes per day.

- *Dyspnoea* occurs in 60%:
  usually disproportionate to the X-ray changes
  on doing a lung scan there is a marked disturbance of ventilation/perfusion due to the tumour compressing the pulmonary artery.
- *Chest pain* occurs in 40%. Two types:
  poorly localized on the side of the tumour
  pleuritic pain which may be due either to secondary infection or to invasion of the pleura by the tumour.
- *Wheezing* occurs in 15%:
  may be localized, and stridor due to tracheal obstruction by tumour can occur.

Metastatic symptoms and signs

Metastases are already present in 70% of patients with symptoms due to bronchial carcinoma. In 30% the metastases are responsible for the initial symptoms.
  In patients with small cell carcinoma, virtually all have overt or occult spread at the time of diagnosis.
  Intrathoracic metastatic manifestations:

- *Recurrent laryngeal palsy*:
  hoarseness of the voice
  a non-explosive cough
  difficulty in expectoration.
- *Obstruction of the superior vena cava* (SVC) – often due to enlarged mediastinal glands (especially right paratracheal) or to compression by the tumour itself. SVC obstruction occurs most commonly with small cell carcinoma.
- *Suggestive symptoms*:
  difficulty in breathing due to stridor
  dysphagia
  blackouts
  severe headache on coughing.
- *Horner's syndrome* – due to involvement of the cervical sympathetic chain; the signs are unilateral:
  small pupil
  partial ptosis
  enophthalmos (eye sunk into socket)
  lack of sweating on that side of face.
- *Chest pain* – due to invasion of the rib by primary or secondary tumour.
- *Brachial neuralgia* – due to involvement of the brachial plexus by an apical (superior sulcus) tumour. Causes pain along the

medial side of the arm (T1 distribution) and wasting of the small muscles of the hand.
- *Pericarditis* – due to direct invasion of the pericardium by the tumour. Leads to:
  precordial pain
  arrhythmias
  cardiac tamponade.

Extrathoracic metastatic involvement:

The main sites affected are:
- Brain – accounts for 10% of extrathoracic symptoms. Presents with headache, fits and focal neurological symptoms/signs.
- Bone – mainly involves ribs, vertebrae, humerus and femur. The presenting symptom is pain.
- Liver – metastases are often silent. Usually found on abdominal examination – firm, irregular liver. Jaundice is not a common presentation.
- Suprarenal glands – rarely causes Addison's disease.

Non-metastatic systemic involvement:

- *Inappropriate secretion of ADH* – diagnosed by finding:
  low serum sodium level
  low plasma osmolality
  high urinary osmolality.
- *Ectopic ACTH syndrome* (less than 1% of patients):
  commonest with small cell carcinoma
  may lead to Cushing's syndrome.
- *Hypercalcaemia* – in about 6% of patients with lung cancer:
  commonest with squamous cell cancer
  usually due to ectopic secretion of parathormone and calcitonin, and less often to direct involvement of the bone marrow by metastases.
- *Neuromyopathies* – 1% to 2% of patients with lung cancer. Types:
  neuromyopathy
  proximal myopathy
  encephalopathy
  cerebellar degeneration syndrome
  myasthenia gravis type of syndrome (Eaton-Lambert syndrome).
  May precede detection of the lung cancer by 6–12 months
  polymyositis.
- *Anaemia* – in about 7% of patients with lung cancer.
  Sometimes, but not always, leuco-erythroblastic.

- *Vascular disorders* – in 1% to 2% of patients. Types:
  thrombophlebitis migrans
  bleeding disorders
  non-bacterial endocarditis.

Skeletal abnormalities:
  clubbing – in over 50% of patients with squamous cell   carcinoma. Less common with adenocarcinoma and rare in   oat
  cell carcinoma
- *Hypertrophic osteoarthropathy* – occurs in about 2% to 3% of
  patients. It presents with swelling of the wrists and ankles, and
  is associated with gross finger clubbing.

What happens?

Unfortunately the prognosis of lung cancer is still very poor with
less than a 10% 5-year survival rate.

The reasons are the early and rapid metastatic spread (it is
estimated that in 70% of cases there are already metastases at first
diagnosis) and ineffective curative therapies.

The mean life expectancy at diagnosis is around 12 months.
Small cell carcinoma disseminates early and life expectancy is 6
months or less; with adenocarcinoma it is 12–18 months;
squamous cell types may live some years.

Surgery is possible in less than one-half of cases, but where it
is successful in removing the growth, the 5-year survival rate is 25%.

The course of lung cancer in most cases is slow deterioration in
general health with loss of weight and strength, and with local
effects causing distressing cough, secondary infection and breathlessness. In about one-quarter, the effects of metastases on vital
organs such as brain, peripheral neuropathies, endocrine system
and skeleton may be more troublesome than the primary growth.

It is a distressful time for the victim and family. The period of
terminal care may extend for months and requires collaborative
care between the practice, particularly the district (home) nursing
team, hospital and hospice (where available).

What to do?

Before discussing management, it is important to re-emphasize
that *most lung cancers are preventable*, and help in avoiding and
giving up smoking is one of the most beneficial services that can
be provided for patients.

General

- Although a practice of 2000 can expect no more than 1 or 2 new cases of lung cancer in a year, nevertheless, its possibility must be considered in middle-aged and elderly patients (males more than females) who present with new persistent respiratory symptoms, general debility or perhaps rather odd features of neurological, psychiatric and rheumatic disorders.
- Early diagnosis is important, not only to offer best chance of surgical 'cure', but also to avoid recriminations and even possible litigation over delayed, missed or erroneous diagnosis.
- Carry out first-line diagnostic procedures (radiology and sputum cytology), but refer all patients for a specialist opinion.
- Have a practice plan or protocol for possible long-term terminal care, and discuss within the practice.
- Ensure regular support and contacts with patient and family.

Diagnosis of bronchial carcinoma

5% of lung cancer is asymptomatic and is diagnosed on routine chest X-ray. The *chest X-ray* is the most useful simple investigation and may show:

- peripheral cancer – average size is 3 cm on diagnosis
- collapse/consolidation with/without a hilar mass
- pleural effusion – these are common and often bloodstained
- diaphragmatic paralysis – due to involvement of the phrenic nerve by the tumour
- hilar and/or mediastinal glands
- lung abscess – due to a necrotic squamous cell cancer.

It is important to identify the cell type and to assess the extent of the process and possibilities for surgery. This involves examination of the sputum for cells, bronchoscopy and CT scan, assessment of local spread and other investigations on the skeleton to exclude metastases.

Sputum cytology results in 40% of cases positive with a single specimen and up to 85% with multiple specimens. More likely to be positive with central lesions than peripheral lesions. The best specimens to examine are those produced in the early morning, and also soon after a bronchoscopy.

Bronchoscopy confirms the diagnosis in over 95% of patients if tumour is visible. Overall positive in 60–70% of cases.

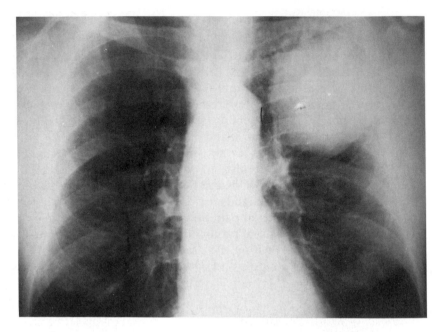

Fig. 12.2(a)—Chest X-ray showing large upper lobe carcinoma on left

Treatment of lung cancer

The main factors influencing treatment are:

- the histological type of the tumour
- stage of the disease and the degree of spread.

Squamous cell carcinoma grows only slowly, tends to remain localized and has the best prognosis.

Small cell carcinoma disseminates early and widely and has the worst prognosis.

Adenocarcinoma and *large cell carcinoma* are intermediate in prognosis.

Types of treatment available

Surgery:

- Best treatment for all carcinomas other than small cell. Squamous cell has the best prognosis.
- 60% of all lung cancers will be found to be inoperable after full investigation.
- Survival at 5 years is 25%; 10 years is 17%.
- Operative mortality – pneumonectomy 6%
               lobectomy 2–4%.

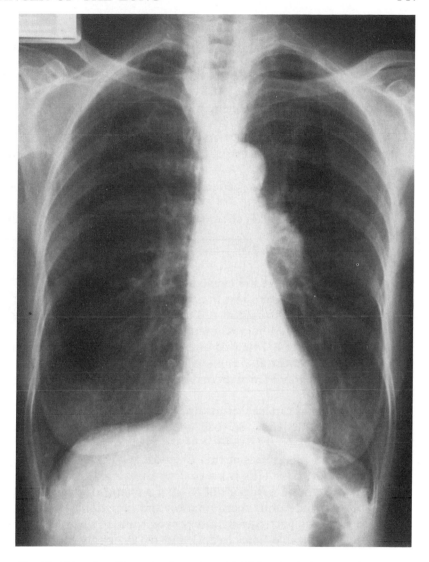

Fig. 12.2(b)—Chest X-ray showing enlarged left hilar glands due to carcinoma

Radiotherapy:

- 5-year survival is similar to surgery in operable cases where there are contra-indications to an operation.
- Post-operative radiation does not improve prognosis.
- Inoperable patients – 5 year survival no more than 10% and the place of radiotherapy in these patients is uncertain.
- Palliative radiotherapy is useful in:

recurrent haemoptysis
persistent pneumonia distal to a bronchial obstruction caused
    by a tumour
obstruction of the superior vena cava by tumour or glands
bone pain
cerebral metastases causing a rise in intracranial pressure.

Cytotoxic treatment:

- Little evidence that cytotoxic drugs improve survival in small cell carcinoma.
- 20% of sensitive lung cancers will show a good initial response, but deteriorate later.
- The value of cyclical chemotherapy still remains to be shown.

Practical points

- Most lung cancers are preventable by not smoking.
- Lung cancer is the most prevalent neoplasm in the UK.
- Annually 40 000 deaths (28 000 men and 12 000 women); deaths in men falling, women's death rates rising.
- GP can expect 1–2 new cases each year and 5 or more patients with lung cancer at various stages in his practice of 2000.
- Lung cancer incidence increases with age, but occurs from age 45 onwards.
- 90% of lung cancer victims are dead within 5 years.
- Prognosis depends on cell type and extent of local and metastatic spread.
- 70% have metastases at first diagnosis.
- First priority for GPs is preventing smoking.
- Early diagnosis is important to offer a chance for surgical cure and to avoid family recrimination and litigation.
- Beware of persistent respiratory symptoms in the middle-aged and inexplicable neurological and psychiatric symptoms and aches and pains.
- Basic GP investigations are chest X-ray and sputum cytology.
- Refer all possible cases for a specialist opinion.
- Surgical excision is possible only in 1 in 4 cases, results are better with 25% 5-year survival.
- Practice plan or protocol for care is necessary and terminal home care by collaboration with district nurses and hospice is important.
- Regular support and explanation to family and patient are essential.

CARDIOVASCULAR DISEASES

CHAPTER 13

CARDIOVASCULAR DISEASES – THE CLINICAL SPECTRUM

Whilst cardiovascular diseases cause almost one-half of all deaths, they make up less than 10% of all consultations. The reasons are that they tend to affect predominantly older persons with national higher mortality rates and relatively fewer consultations for each episode.

Patient consulting rates

Composite data from the Third National Morbidity Survey (1981–2) and J.F.'s experience (Table 13.1) shows that 12% of all persons will consult in a year for cardiovascular diagnoses. The diagnostic range is wide, including life-threatening acute myocardial infarctions to minor varicose veins and their local complications.

TABLE 13.1 Annual consulting rates for cardiovascular diseases

Condition	per 2000	per 10 000
IHD		
Acute myocardial infarction	8	40
Angina	14	70
Chronic ischaemic heart disease	14	70
Total	36	180
Arrhythmias	10	50
Heart failure	24	120
Peripheral vascular diseases	9	45
Varicose veins	19	95
Phlebitis and thrombosis	8	40
Haemorrhoids	17	85
Total	44	220
High blood pressure	100	500
Anaemia	20	100
(Pernicious anaemia)	(3)	(15)
Other vascular	2	10

Cardiovascular diseases make up 10% of all consultations. Most are for management of high blood pressure and ischaemic heart disease.

Sickness/invalidity benefits

These are benefits for 'workers', that is persons between 16 and 65. Cardiovascular diagnoses have made up 17% of days certified by GPs for absence from work. IHD, high blood pressure and 'other heart diseases' were the main causes of sickness/invalidity (OHE, 1986).

Hospital in-patient data

Surprisingly only 6.7% of 'discharges and deaths' were for cardiovascular diseases (Health and Personal Social Services Statistics,

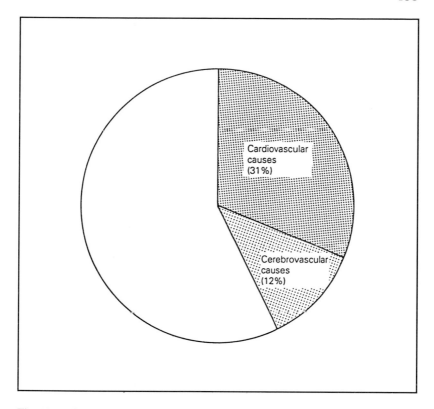

Fig. 13.1—Cardiovascular diseases cause almost one-half of all deaths

1991) (males 8.2% and females 5.4%). It appears that most persons with cardiovascular diseases are treated in the community and out-patient departments.

Causes of death

As noted (pages 10) cardiac and cerebral vascular diseases account for almost one-half (43%) of all certified deaths in the UK.

Out of 600 000 deaths (1990):
Cardiovascular causes were   31%
Cerebrovascular   12%
   (OHE 1992)

CHAPTER 14

HIGH BLOOD PRESSURE

What is it?

The diagnosis of high blood pressure is essentially an exercise in measurement. It is one of the few conditions whose label is applied as a result, almost entirely, of an objective measurement by a man-made machine – the sphygmomanometer.

The diagnosis and management of high blood pressure requires a careful mix of art and science – the art of selective discrimination applied to the personal needs of the patient, plus the science learned from experience and academic research. Science based on sphygmomanometric readings must not be allowed to overrule the art of personal care.

What level is 'abnormal' or 'diseased'? This is based on what blood pressure levels lead to adverse effects on other organs, such as the heart, lungs and kidneys. Life insurance companies base their premiums on 140/90. Clinical studies in the past have usually assessed diastolic pressure levels only, and the results have shown that diastolic levels above 100 mm can lead to long-term adverse effects on these organs; therefore, this level has been regarded in the UK as the relevant one at which treatment should be considered. More recent studies have indicated that systolic pressure levels are equally important in determining prognosis, but as yet there is insufficient evidence from appropriate clinical trials to help in deciding how to best deal with systolic hypertension.

Such rigid mensural definitions of a disease are unhelpful in practice, when we do not know or understand the true causes, course and outcome of most cases of so-called high blood pressure.

High blood pressure and its understanding provide an excellent example of the need for flexibility of approach and thought if we are to manage our patients satisfactorily and with the least anxiety and discomfort.

It is likely that blood pressure levels represent a graded multi-factorial human characteristic, like height and weight, rather than a specific disease associated with a single gene with its incomplete dominance. However, the situation is complicated by the fact that there are definite genetic associations. For example, if both parents are hypertensive then the offspring stand a 50% chance of having high blood pressure and if one parent is hypertensive the chances of offspring being hypertensive are 25%.

A condition that affects up to 20% of all adults cannot readily be classified as a 'disease', unless and until the natural history is known and the outcome related to a variety of factors.

High blood pressure increases with age and is more frequent in females than in males. The course and outcome are related to age, sex, level of blood pressure and family history. The challenge must be to pick out the vulnerable persons who require life-long care and treatment and not to subject as many as 1 in 5 of the adult population, in whom the prognosis may be good, to the miseries of medication.

High blood pressure becomes a 'disease' when its effects produce organ damage in the heart, brain, eyes and kidneys, and the aim of management must be to prevent such damage from taking place.

At the present state of knowledge three varieties of high blood pressure are recognized:

(1) *Primary or essential benign hypertension* where no underlying causes are found
(2) *Secondary hypertension* (see also pages 166)
   • *Renal disease* – commonest cause
     chronic infection, e.g. pyelonephritis
     chronic nephritis
     renal artery stenosis
     polycystic disease
     hydronephrosis
   • *Endocrine disease*
     Conn's syndrome (primary hyperaldosteronism)
     Cushing's syndrome

phaeochromocytoma
- *Coarctation of the aorta*
- *Drugs (iatrogenic)*
contraceptive pill
post-menopausal hormone replacement therapy
steroids
non-steroidal anti-inflammatory drugs

(3) Malignant, namely a very high level of blood pressure with progressive complications and rapid death in untreated cases.

In practice 90% of hypertensives are benign and essentially of unknown cause, 5% are malignant and 5% are secondary to some definable, and often treatable, cause.

We are at a stage, therefore, of having to manage a condition characterized by a higher than 'normal' blood pressure, a condition of unknown cause in the majority of cases and uncertain outcome, a condition where the raised blood pressure can be controlled by drugs with side-effects that may be unpleasant and which may have to be taken for the rest of the person's life.

General practitioners need to be careful in basing their management of hypertension on hospital practice. Patients referred to hospital for hypertension are almost inevitably those with severe hypertension which is difficult to control, patients with secondary hypertension possibly requiring surgical treatment or those with target organ complications, such as renal failure or heart failure. This type of patient is certainly not representative of the hypertensive patients seen in general practice.

Who has it and when?

Apart from its clinical implications as a potential extra risk for stroke and cardiovascular diseases, the other major problem is the high rate of 'high blood pressure' in the community.

Using the figure of 140/90 as upper limit of normal then the rates in the community are:

- 10–15% of the whole population
- 20% of all over 40s
- 30% of all over 65s
- 40% of all over 75s

Translated to a general practice with 2000 patients it means that there are likely to be up to 300 persons with blood pressure over

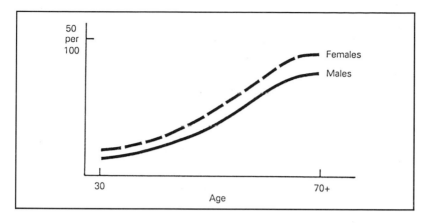

Fig. 14.1—Frequency of hypertension in over-30s

140/90 but at present less than one-half will be known and under care. The numbers will be:

- *up to 300 per 2000 patients*
- 150 of those aged 40–64
- 100 of those aged 65–74
- 50 of those over 75

Such numbers reveal the potential amount of care that may be required for long-term management in the community and in general practice.

High blood pressure is a condition associated with *ageing* – the age prevalence increases with each decade and is higher in females than males (Figure 14.1).

On grading high blood pressure into mild, moderate and severe by levels of diastotic blood pressure (DBP), most (85%) are mild (Figure 14.2).

	Mild	Moderate	Severe
DBP	90–109	110–129	130+
%	85	13.5	1.5

In addition to age there are other related factors:

- sex – higher in females
- family – genetic influences

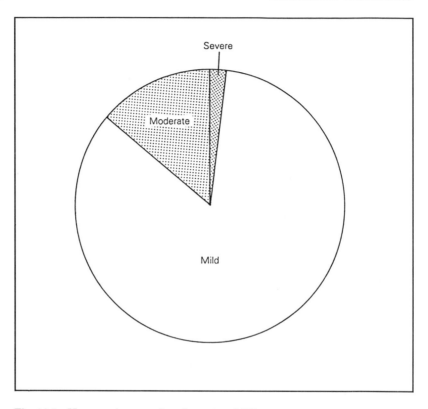

Fig. 14.2—Hypertension – grades of severity of GP cases

- culture – higher in urbanized societies
- race – lower in Africans and Japanese and higher in American negroes
- obesity – higher
- alcoholics – higher
- social class – higher in 5 than 1.

Malignant hypertension

Although rare in general practice, occurring about once every ten years, it is a very serious condition with very high blood pressure levels – 250 + /140 +, accompanied by haematuria, renal failure and grade 3/4 hypertensive retinopathy. If left untreated, the condition is almost always fatal as a result of heart failure, renal failure or stroke. It is controllable by appropriate drug treatment,

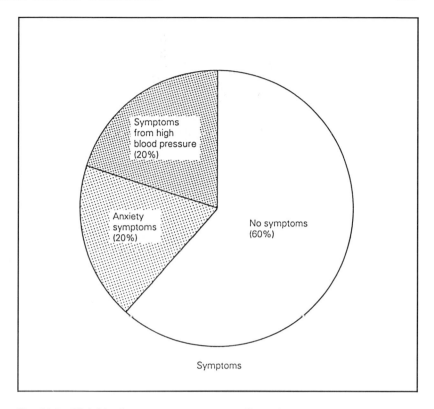

Fig. 14.3—High blood pressure – symptoms at diagnosis

and constitutes a medical emergency requiring immediate hospital admission.

How does it present?

The majority of persons found to have high blood pressure have no symptoms. The finding of a raised blood pressure is being increasingly discovered on routine examination of apparently 'well' persons.

60% of newly discovered hypertensives have no symptoms, 20% anxiety symptoms that may not be related to high blood pressure and 20% have symptoms that may have been associated with an awareness of raised blood pressure.

- *Headache* – only with very high levels of blood pressure – say $250+/130+$. Most headaches occurring in patients with

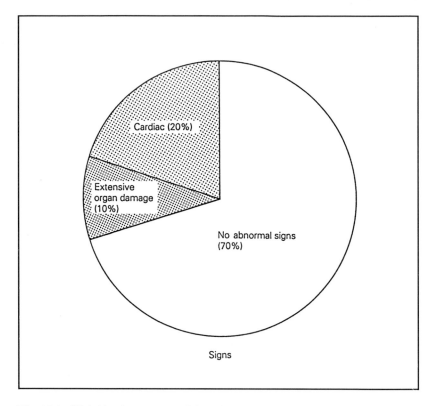

Fig. 14.4—High blood pressure – clinical signs at diagnosis

hypertension are due to anxiety. Hypertensive headache tends
to be occipital, throbbing, worse on waking and lasting for hours.
- *Troublesome nose bleeds* are frequent in elderly persons with high
  blood pressure but they are also frequent in those with normal
  blood pressure, probably due to sclerotic nasal blood vessels.

Other symptoms associated with the complications of high blood
pressure include:

- dizziness – carotid and cerebral arterial disease
- angina – coronary artery disease
- breathlessness – due to hypertensive left ventricular failure
- claudication – peripheral artery disease
- visual deterioration – retinal vascular disease
- symptoms due to hypertensive renal failure such as polyuria,
  loss of weight, anaemia.

There are no specific signs of high blood pressure itself, apart from the levels. Signs that may be found are those of complications (Figure 14.4):

- 70% no abnormal complications;
- 20% evidence of cardiac strain;
- 10% retinopathy, renal abnormalities or after-effects of strokes.

Signs are more prominent in secondary hypertension and are illustrated in Figure 14.5.

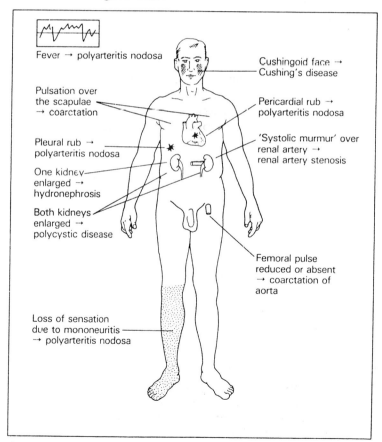

Fever → polyarteritis nodosa

Pulsation over the scapulae → coarctation

Pleural rub → polyarteritis nodosa

One kidney enlarged → hydronephrosis

Both kidneys enlarged → polycystic disease

Cushingoid face → Cushing's disease

Pericardial rub → polyarteritis nodosa

'Systolic murmur' over renal artery → renal artery stenosis

Femoral pulse reduced or absent → coarctation of aorta

Loss of sensation due to mononeuritis → polyarteritis nodosa

Fig. 14.5—Possible clinical signs in secondary hypertension

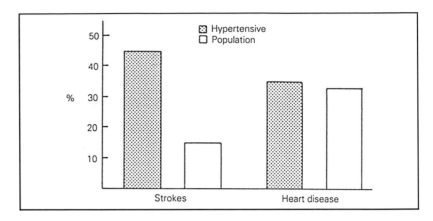

Fig. 14.6—Death rates from strokes and heart disease – comparison of hypertensives with the general population

What happens?

In deciding on management that may involve medication for 30 years or more it is of particular importance to understand the likely *natural history, course, outcome and risks of complications.*

The majority of mild hypertensives probably have normal life expectancies with no complications, even if untreated.

- High blood pressure does increase risk of developing a stroke 2 or 3-fold (Figure 14.6).
- High blood pressure does *not* increase risk of coronary heart disease.

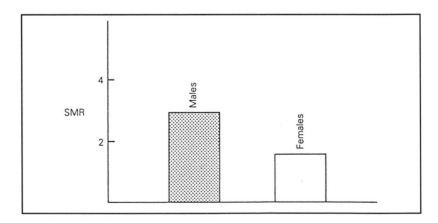

Fig. 14.7—Hypertensives – mortality risks twice as high in males as in females

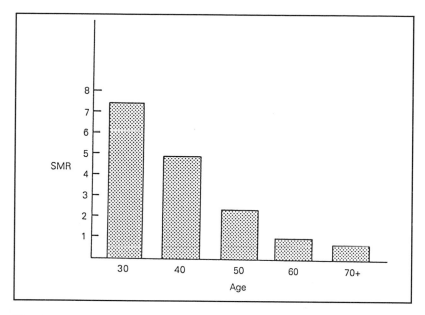

Fig. 14.8—Hypertensives – inverse relationship of mortality rates and age at diagnosis

- High blood pressure does increase risk of premature death, in younger hypertensives.

  There are some definable *risk factors* of *outcome*:

- mortality rates higher in males (Figure 14.7);

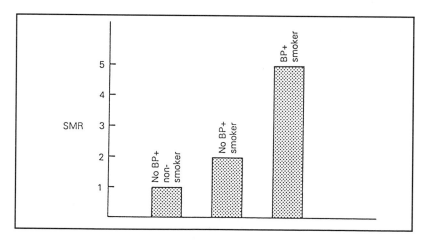

Fig. 14.9—Smoking is an added mortality risk factor in hypertension

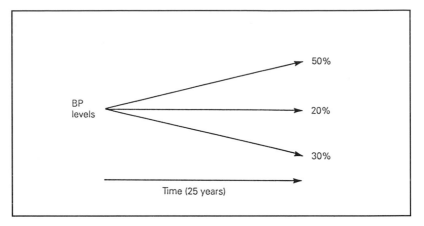

Fig. 14.10—Blood pressure levels do not inevitably rise with age

- *age* at diagnosis with risks appreciably higher in younger hypertensives (Figure 14.8);
- *family history* of early deaths from strokes and heart attacks increases risk 3-fold;
- *smokers* with high blood pressure have extra risks (Figure 14.9);
- the higher the *blood pressure levels* the greater the risks of mortality and complications.

The *benefits* of *treatment* have to be critically evaluated. Whilst large trials of results of treating hypertensives at all ages do show 'statistically significant' benefits in reduction of strokes, nevertheless, there is no convincing evidence of reductions in overall mortality or deaths from coronary artery disease.

However, these benefits are by no means universal or absolute. It is important to have some idea of the size of any benefits in relation to the amount, extent and duration of treatment necessary to prevent one stroke or one coronary event.

A measure is to calculate the number of 'patient-years' (i.e. a length of time) of treatment that is required to prevent a single stroke and a single coronary event. This has been done by Beard Katal (Management of elderly patients with sustained hypertension, *British Medical Journal*, 1992, 304, 412–6).

They show that:

- in *younger hypertensives* (aged 40–64) treatment for 833 patient-years is required to prevent one stroke and there is no benefit on prevention of a coronary event.
- in *older hypertensives* (aged 65–75) treatment for 370 patient-

years is required to prevent one stroke and treatment for 417 patient-years to prevent one coronary event.

Put another way – how many hypertensives need to be treated for 30 years in the younger group of 40–64 and for 10 years in the older group of 65–75?

- 28 hypertensives (aged 40–64) need to be treated for 30 years to prevent one stroke.
- 37 elderly hypertensives (aged 65–75) need to be treated for 10 years to prevent one stroke and 42 to prevent one coronary event.

Such data demands that a balance of common sense is struck in decisions on long-term medication.

What to do?

Assessment

There are many problems and difficulties in coming to a reasonable assessment of each patient with raised blood pressure.

Our approach will be made easier and more sensitive if the following points are taken into account.

1. *Is there 'high blood pressure'?*

It has to be proven that there is a persistently raised blood pressure of significant levels to merit a diagnosis of 'high blood pressure'. A single random and casual reading is inadequate and at least three separate recordings should be taken and all should show raised levels before labelling the patient as 'hypertensive'. These three blood pressures should be taken *at intervals of at least one month* as one-half of patients diagnosed as hypertensive can settle spontaneously.

Due consideration must be given to the age, sex and family history in translating the sphygmomanometric figures into a permanent diagnostic label that will haunt patient and physician.

2. *Is there any underlying cause?*

The possibility, albeit an unusual one, must be considered of high blood pressure being secondary to some causal disease. Although less than 5% of hypertensives have some definite underlying cause a search should be undertaken in all younger patients. Younger hypertensives are more likely to have remediable, though rare, causes.

The mnemonic CASSIUS suggests possible remediable causes of high blood pressure:

- Coarctation of the aorta
- Aldosteronism (Conn's syndrome)
- Suprarenal diseases such as phaeochromocytoma and Cushing's syndrome
- Stenosis of a renal artery
- Infection and inflammation of the kidneys in chronic pyalonephritis and chronic nephritis
- Unilateral kidney disease apart from renal artery stenosis
- Steroid drugs causing iatrogenic hypertension.

The history may help in distinguishing primary and secondary hypertension:

- Is there any family history of hypertension – common in primary hypertension?
- Any past history or current symptoms of renal disease, commonest cause of secondary hypertension?
- Any treatment with drugs, e.g. NSAIDs, contraceptive pill, steroids.

3. *What is the probable natural course?*

The course of the hypertension will depend on: (see pages 162–4)

- age and sex – younger patients and males far worse
- height of the blood pressure – the systolic level is likely to be as significant as the diastolic
- family history of premature death from hypertension, coronary disease or stroke will affect the prognosis adversely
- presence of complications affecting the target organs – heart, kidneys and brain
- presence of associated risk factors:
  cigarette smoking
  raised blood cholesterol
  diabetes
  obesity.

It should not be assumed that a raised blood pressure in an individual will persist for ever or increase with age.

Observations in J.F.'s practice (Figure 14.10) revealed that in a follow-up over 25 years:

- in 50% it went up
- in 20% it stayed the same
- in 30% it went down.

Spontaneous fall in blood pressure may occur:

- following a major myocardial infarction
- following left ventricular failure
- in some elderly persons
- sometimes after raised blood pressure with good control using antihypertensive drugs, the blood pressure will remain normal when drugs are withdrawn. We should be prepared to cease drug treatment at times to see if the blood pressure will remain at normal levels without therapy.

4. *What are the side-effects of therapy?*

It should be appreciated just what specific treatment entails for the individual patient. It means life-long supervision and medication with potent drugs with possible unpleasant side-effects.

5. *GP investigation*

The purpose is largely to help in deciding the prognosis. This will depend primarily on involvement of target organs as a result of the hypertension. The tests which may be of value to the GP in this respect are:

- urine examination – for proteinuria and haematuria;
- chest X-ray for cardiac enlargement (the X-ray gives no information about whether left ventricular *hypertrophy* is present);
- ECG – this is the test for deciding left ventricular hypertrophy. The other possible relevant finding is evidence of myocardial ischaemia, e.g. an old myocardial infarction;
- blood urea – a raised blood urea level is a good indication of established renal failure. A more sensitive test for picking up early renal impairment is the blood creatinine level.

Tests for secondary hypertension are usually carried out by the hospital team.

Management of hypertension

The aims of management are:

- reduction in mortality
- less left ventricular failure
- less chance of stroke, especially haemorrhagic
- reduced risk of renal failure.

Which patients should be treated right away?

- Malignant hypertension

BP 250+/140+
grade 3/4 retinopathy
haematuria/renal failure
- Target organ damage
heart → angina, left ventricular failure
brain → stroke, TIAs
kidneys → raised blood urea

Which patients should be treated but not so urgently?

- Blood pressure levels diastolic over 100 mm (persistent) – systolic levels uncertain (further trial evidence required).
- Younger patients under 55 years of age.
- Males would weigh the balance for treatment.
- Bad family history.
- Black patients – have a worse prognosis with hypertension.
- Presence of other risk factors as above.

Which patients probably do not need treatment?

- Labile hypertension – continue regular observation only.
- Elderly patients (over 65) with mild hypertension below 180/110.
- Females with mild hypertension and no other adverse factors.
- Obese patients – try weight reduction first.
- Mild hypertension (not above 160/100) and no other risk factors or adverse family history.

(Note: 85% of hypertensives are mild).

Treatment of hypertension

Having made a careful decision to treat them consider following:

General

- *Control risk factors*
  smoking
  high blood cholesterol (especially in the young)
  diabetes
  stop contraceptive pill
  reduce weight if obese.
- *Reduce salt intake* – to no more than about 3 g/day which means no added salt at table.
- *Reduce alcohol consumption.*
- *Regular enjoyable non-competitive exercise.*

Specific drug treatment

The main groups of drugs available are:

- diuretics, e.g. thiazides
- calcium-channel blockers, e.g. nifedipine, verapamil
- beta-blockers, e.g. atenolol
- angiotensin-converting enzyme inhibitors (ACEI), e.g. captopril, enalapril
- peripheral vasodilators, e.g. prazosin, minoxidil.

Thiazides: Although thiazides are often used as first-line treatment, they are not always effective alone and may also lead to side-effects:

- hyperglycaemia with exacerbation of diabetes
- hypokalaemia → excessive fatigue
- hyperuricaemia → precipitation of gout
- impotence in young males
- adverse effects on blood lipids – though the clinical significance of this remains to be shown.

Calcium-channel blockers: These drugs act mainly by producing peripheral vasodilatation, but some may also reduce the force of cardiac contraction. They can be very effective in lowering blood pressure but may also produce uncomfortable side-effects:

- flushing and feelings of heat, especially nifedipine
- ankle swelling – again mainly with nifedipine
- palpitations
- constipation, especially verapamil
- postural dizziness, especially in the elderly with cerebrovascular insufficiency.

Beta-blockers: These drugs are often effective and are especially useful in hypertensive patients who also have angina. In practice their use is often limited by contraindications and side-effects:

- associated asthma or chronic obstructive lung disease – there is a tendency to bronchospasm with the beta-blockers, even if they are designated cardiospecific, e.g. atenolol
- claudication – peripheral vasospasm may aggravate this condition
- excessive fatigue – this is more common with beta-blockers than generally realized
- early heart failure can be exacerbated
- sleep disturbances – especially with propranolol

- impotence
- adverse effects on blood lipids – increase in the level of triglyceride and reduction in level of HDL-cholesterol (which *inhibits atherosclerosis*).

ACEI: There are very effective drugs in hypertension and are being used more frequently now as first-line treatment. Care must be taken when giving the first dose as this may occasionally cause a significant fall of standing blood pressure associated with postural dizziness. This is more likely to occur in patients who are on potent diuretic treatment for heart failure – this causes a high level of circulating angiotensin which helps to maintain the blood pressure in these patients; a sudden fall in angiotensin levels induced by ACEIs may therefore result in a precipitous fall in blood pressure. In view of this potential reaction to ACEI it is always advisable to start treatment with a small dose and check the standing blood pressure fall before embarking on regular treatment with the standard dose.

There are a few other adverse effects with these drugs:

- cough;
- renal impairment – but only in those patients whose renal function is already impaired, and only with high doses
- neutropenia – a rare side-effect and also usually with high doses of the ACEI. It is more likely to occur in patients who may already be immuno-suppressed, e.g. AIDS, treated malignancy.

Peripheral vasodilators: These drugs act directly on the arterial wall producing vasodilatation and a fall in blood pressure. The main hazard with this group of drugs is in causing too large a fall of standing blood pressure resulting in postural dizziness; this is especially prone to occur in elderly patients who have cerebrovascular disease.

Drugs in this group include:

- Prazosin, terazosin – the difficulty with these drugs is the large dose range which may make the initial dose titration unduly prolonged.
- Hydralazine – this is an effective drug but carries the significant risk of developing a syndrome like systemic lupus erythematosus.
- Minoxidil – again an effective drug but with significant side-effects, e.g. fluid retention and hirsutism in women.
- Methyl dopa (Aldomet) – this is a good old-fashioned drug which may still be useful in controlling hypertension, especially in those patients who cannot take any of the previous drugs for

whatever contraindications or who have unacceptable side-effects. It acts centrally and reduces sympathetic activity on the blood vessels, thereby leading to vasodilatation. Side-effects may occur but are infrequent – they include drowsiness, fatigue, bowel disturbances and impotence.

Resistant hypertension

This can be a problem and usually requires hospital referral. However, it is worth checking a few of the possible causes first, which, if present, may remove the need for referral:

- The obvious first possibility is not taking the drugs.
- Exclude other drug treatment which may be inhibiting the response to the hypertensive treatment:
  NSAIDs
  steroids
  oestrogens, e.g. 'the pill', hormone replacement therapy in post-menopausal women
  don't forget over-the-counter medicines which the patient may be taking unknown to the GP, e.g. ibuprofen, sympathomimetic cold remedies, nasal sprays, etc.
- Try adding a loop diuretic, e.g. frusemide, bumetanide, as fluid retention is common with hypotensive drugs and may be inhibiting the hypotensive effects.
- An inadequate dose of the hypotensive drug may have been prescribed. Always try the maximum dose of the drug as recommended in the BNF if the patient can tolerate it.

In J.F.'s practice resistant (poorly controlled) hypertension occurred in 20% of all those treated and only moderately good control (DBP 90–109 mm) in another 20%.

Planned care

With such large numbers of hypertensives to be managed, effectively good planning is necessary at a number of levels:

- Each practice should devise its own agreed protocols and guidelines.
- Shared care arranged between nurse and doctor.
- Continuity of personal care important.
- Early diagnosis, either opportunistic at routine consultation or screening (aim to measure and record blood pressure of adults over 40 every 5 years).

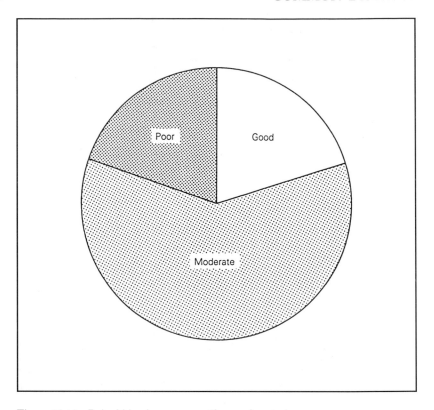

Figure 14.11—Raised blood pressure – efficacy of control

- Management assessment is responsibility of doctor.
- Those on treatment, once controlled, should be seen at set intervals by nurse or doctor during normal consultations or at special mini-clinics.
- Doctor should see the patient at least once a year as part of audit exercise.
- Collaboration between GPs and local hospital specialist is important, particularly in drawing up guidelines for referral.

Practical points

- High blood pressure is a disease diagnosed by a machine, the sphygmomanometer.
- Causes are uncertain in 90% of 'primary essential hypertension'.
- Risks associated with high blood pressure are strokes, left ventricular failure, renal failure and premature death.
- However, most mild hypertensives have normal life expectancies with no complications.
- Particular at-risk groups are younger (under 60s), males more than females, family history of strokes and heart attacks and high levels of blood pressure.
- Most hypertension is mild (85%), with moderate 13.5% and severe 1.5%.
- Major problem of care is the high prevalence – 20% of over 40-year-olds are hypertensive and 40% of over 75s.
- No specific symptoms, clinical assessment is based on detection of any organ damage of heart, kidneys and eyes.
- Aims of management are to reduce overall mortality, prevent strokes, left ventricular failure and renal failure and to make the long-term treatment acceptable for the patient.
- However, it requires lots of preventive medication – in under 65s treatment for 833 patient-years and in over 65s 370 patient-years to prevent 1 stroke.
- Management of such large numbers of hypertensives, up to 300 per GP with 2000 patients, demands planned care with agreed practice protocols and guidelines developed in collaboration with local hospital specialists; shared care between practice nurses and doctors; early diagnosis through opportunistic and screening methods; first clinical assessment by doctor and then at least once a year.
- General measures such as stopping smoking, reduction of overweight, control of alcohol, reduction of salt intake and regular exercise should precede specific medication.
- Specific measures involve step by step medication with diuretics, calcium channel blockers, beta-blockers, angiotensin converter enzyme inhibitors, peripheral vasodilators.
- Although good control is obtained in 60%, some 20% are 'resistant' and may require referral to a specialist.

CHAPTER **15**

ISCHAEMIC HEART DISEASE

What is it?

Ischaemic heart disease (IHD) is a collective term for local cardiac manifestations of atherosclerosis, a generalized body disorder.

Causes of atherosclerosis are uncertain but it is associated with ageing and there are certain *risk factors*.

Risk factors

Major
- hypertension
- hypercholesterolaemia
- smoking

Other
- family history of premature deaths from IHD
- diabetes
- obesity
- oral contraceptives (especially in smokers)
- soft water

Doubtful
- lack of exercise
- mental stress
- dietary – too much sugar

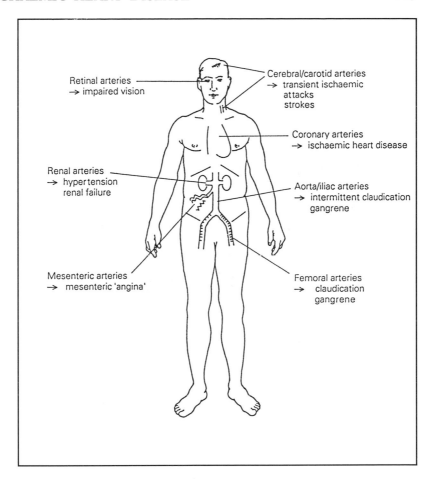

Retinal arteries
→ impaired vision

Cerebral/carotid arteries
→ transient ischaemic
   attacks
   strokes

Coronary arteries
→ ischaemic heart disease

Renal arteries
→ hypertension
   renal failure

Aorta/iliac arteries
→ intermittent claudication
   gangrene

Mesenteric arteries
→ mesenteric 'angina'

Femoral arteries
→ claudication
   gangrene

Fig. 15.1—Clinical effects of atherosclerosis associated with hypertension

The predominant *clinical effects* of atherosclerosis depend on the arteries affected.

- Coronary arteries – ischaemic heart disease.
- Cerebral and carotid – strokes and transient ichaemic attacks.
- Retinal – retinopathy.
- Renal and aorta – hypertension and renal failure.
- Aorta and mesenteric – mesenteric angina and intestinal ischaemia.
- Iliac and femoral – claudication.

It should be noted that a person with one clinical disorder also is prone to ischaemic changes at other sites.

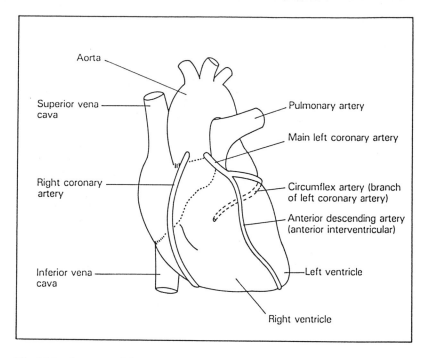

Fig. 15.2—Anatomy of the coronary arteries

Coronary arteries

The main coronary arteries are:

- left main stem and left anterior descending
- circumflex branch (of left coronary)
- right coronary.

Prognosis depends on the extent and site of atherosclerotic occlusion. Thus occlusion of:

- left main stem – 20% mortality per year
- other single vessel – 1–2% mortality per year
- 2 vessels – 6% mortality per year
- 3 vessels – 10% mortality per year.

General trends

IHD is the largest single cause of death – 27% of overall deaths (33% of all deaths in males and 25% of all deaths in females).

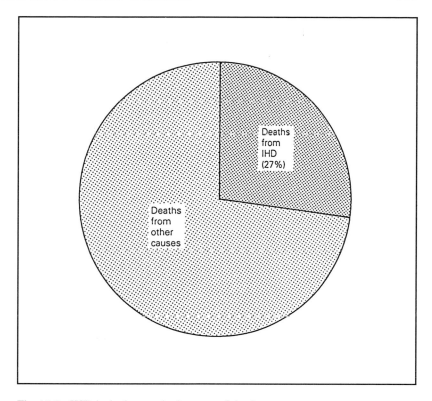

Fig. 15.3—IHD is the largest single cause of death

Over the past 10 years there have been falls in deaths from IHD in many developed countries:

- USA and Australia reduction by 30%
- UK reduction by 19% in men and 15% in women
- West Germany and Sweden reduction by less than 10%.

Who gets what and when?

It is likely that there are around ½ million new cases of IHD a year in the UK and over 1 million under care by GPs.

Incidence rises progressively with *age* and it is *more frequent in men than women* but the difference is decreasing because of decline in men and increase in women.

The *clinical spectrum* of IHD in general practice is shown in Table 15.1. For a GP with 2000 patients there will be 40 with IHD and for a group with 10 000 some 200 IHD patients.

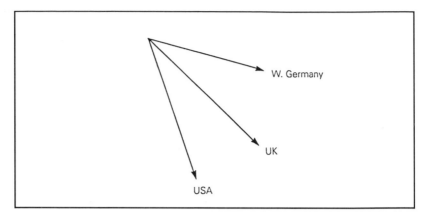

Fig. 15.4—Falling death rates from IHD in last 10 years: USA down 30%; UK down 19% in men, 15% in women; West Germany down less than 10%

The proportions of various clinical types are:

- myocardial infarction (acute)   30%
- angina   35%
- chronic IHD   30%
- other   5%

TABLE 15.1   Annual consultation rates for IHD

Condition	per 2000	per 10 000
Acute myocardial infarction (MI)	12	60
(Sudden death)	(4)	(20)
Angina	14	70
Chronic (heart failure, post MI, arrhythmias and other)	14	70
Total	40	200

The *sex differences* for each category were for myocardial infarction M : F = 2 : 1 and for the other two categories M : F = 4 : 3, thus more men suffer from the acute forms of IHD.

What happens?

As already noted, IHD is the largest single cause of death in the

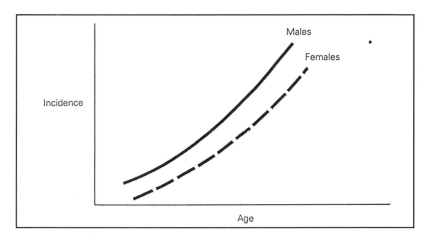

Fig. 15.5—Incidence of IHD rises progressively with age and is more frequent in men than in women

UK – 160 000 deaths or 5 per GP (2000 patients), 25 per practice (10 000 patients), annually.

Angina

The proportion who die in 5 years after diagnosis is 20% (compared with 12% expected deaths). One-half have minor or no symptoms easily controlled by changes in lifestyles or medication. However, 30% have considerable disability and 10% will be severely disabled (Table 15.2).

TABLE 15.2 Angina patients – 5-year prognosis

Outcome	%
Dead	20 (worse for unstable angina)
No symptoms or controlled without medication	15
Symptoms well controlled with medication	35
Moderate control with medication (disability +)	20
Severe symptoms (disability ++)	10

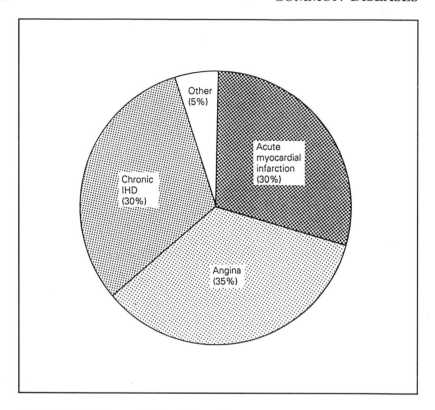

Fig. 15.6—Clinical types of ischaemic heart disease

It is the 30% with moderate–severe disability who are candidates for *angiography and possible surgery*.

Note again that annual deaths are related to vessels occluded:

1 vessel   – 1–2% death risk
2 vessels   –   6% death risk
3 vessels   – 10% death risk
L. main stem – 20% death risk

Myocardial infarction

After 5 years almost one-half are dead (including the sudden deaths within 24 hours of onset).

However, of those patients who survive for 1 week after the acute episode, 75% will be alive 5 years later.

TABLE 15.3 Myocardial infarction – outcome

Outcome	%
Dead	45
No symptoms and no disability	15
Moderate disability	20
Severe disability	20

What to do?

Aims   The general aims are:

Clinical

- To save and prolong life.
- To improve and maintain cardiac function.
- To relieve symptoms.
- To prevent complications.

Prevention

- To endeavour to prevent or delay onset and development of
  atherosclerosis.
- In childhood:
  breast-feeding – less sugar, fat, salt
  avoid excessive weight gain
  weaning – limit saturated fat, avoid added sugar and salt
  review school meals
  encourage regular exercise
  discourage smoking
  (remember familial hypercholesterolaemia).
- Young adults:
  DISCOURAGE SMOKING
  control overweight
  avoid excess fat, high cholesterol foods
  regular *enjoyable* exercise.
- Established (symptomatic disease):
  look for risk factors:
      smoking
      hypertension
      high cholesterol
      diabetes

oral contraception
obesity
encourage regular and *enjoyable* exercise.

Social aims

- To discuss the *personal and family* problems that arise from diagnosis of IHD.
- Lifestyle (as noted).
- Occupation – possible changes (if feasible).
- Regular support from the practice team.
- Arrangements for long-term care and supervision.

Angina

Diagnosis

The diagnosis of angina is made primarily on a careful analysis of the history, especially the characteristics of the *chest pain*.

- *Site*
  classically central behind the sternum
  sometimes left side of chest
  less often right side of chest
  occasionally back of chest
- *Radiation*
  typically across both sides of chest
  left arm very common
  right arm sometimes
  both arms occasionally
  throat and jaw common
  through to back rarely
  down to epigastrium almost never
- *Character* – suggestive features described by patient:
  gripping
  squeezing
  crushing
  'like a vice'
  'like a tight band'
- *Duration:*
  angina lasts for *minutes* (5–10)
  never 'seconds'
  never 'hours' (consider unstable angina and MI)
- *Precipitating factors:*
  exertion

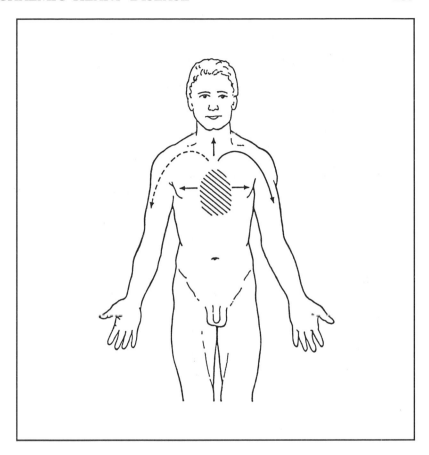

Fig. 15.7—Angina – site and radiation of the pain

emotional stress
cold wind (walking)
heavy meal
● *relief*:
glyceryl trinitrate (within 2 minutes)
stopping exertion
● *Associated symptoms*:
'choking'
'strangling'
'suffocation'
'fighting for breath'
'belching' at end of attack

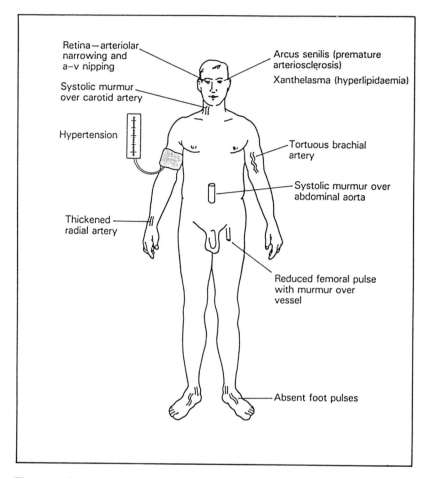

Fig. 15.8—Signs of atherosclerosis

Examination

There are no specific signs of angina but there may be associated features of general atherosclerosis.

Differential diagnosis

The diagnosis of angina may be easy with classical symptoms but the following causes of chest discomfort must be considered:

• anxiety (functional pain)
• pleuritic

- hiatus hernia – oesophagitis
- peptic ulcer and non ulcer dyspepsia
- cervical spondylosis

Investigation

Resting ECG is of limited value unless taken during an attack, but it may show evidence of previous MI.

The exercise test in angina

This is the most useful simple test in angina to pick out those patients who are most likely to benefit from coronary surgery and access to exercise ECG testing should now be available to general practitioners as a screening test.

The presence of ischaemic changes in leads V1–V6 of the ECG *during exercise* (Figure 15.9) suggests the likelihood of disease of the left coronary artery, and the combination of these changes with changes in III, aVF indicates the possibility of multivessel disease; in both of these cases consideration should be given to the desirability of coronary arteriography as the next step.

General measures (check list)

- stop smoking
- control raised blood pressure
- reduce obesity
- correct any anaemia
- reduce hypercholesterolaemia in young (under 50)
- lifestyle and social conditions
- arrangements for long-term care by the practice team

Specific treatment of angina

- *Nitrates*:
  for control of acute attacks – sublingual tablet/spray of glyceryl trinitrate
  for prophylaxis prior to exercise – tablet or spray of GT – use freely
  for long-term prevention – sorbide nitrate up to 120 mg daily.
- *Calcium-channel blockers* – these have superseded beta-blockers as second-line treatment for angina. The advantages over beta-blockers are:
  no peripheral vasoconstriction
  no tendency to bronchospasm
  no adverse effects in diabetes
  no adverse effects on blood lipids

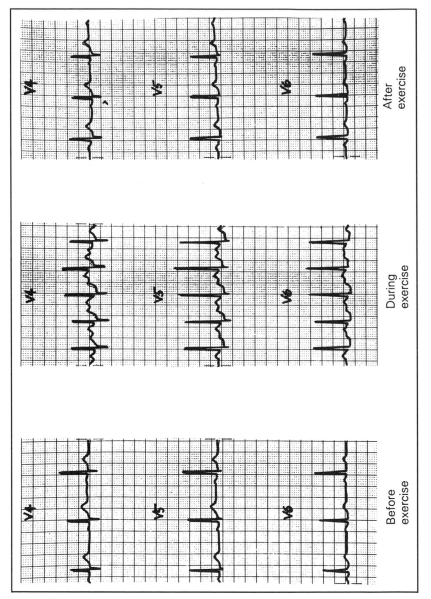

Fig. 15.9—Exercise ECG showing ischaemic S–T depression during exercise

may produce coronary vasodilation (beta-blockers may vasoconstrict the coronary arteries).

Calcium-channel blockers are especially valuable in the treatment of rest (unstable) angina. The drug of choice is probably diltiazem (Tildiem) – it avoids the flushing, oedema and postural hypotension of nifedipine, and also the uncomfortable constipation of verapamil.

- *Beta-blockers*: These drugs still play an important part in the treatment of angina, providing patients with chronic lung disease, diabetes, and intermittent claudication are avoided. The adverse effects on blood lipids remains to be shown to be of any clinical significance.

When should the GP refer a patient with angina to the cardiologist at the local hospital?

- Young patients under 50. The reason for this is that patients with angina due to disease of the left coronary artery or multivessel disease would stand a better chance of survival with coronary surgery than with medical treatment. Although, it would therefore be desirable to investigate all anginal patients with this in mind, the limited resources preclude this option. It is reasonable to concentrate the resources on younger patients.
- Family history of premature death from ischaemic heart disease.
- When angina remains intractable after full medical treatment with nitrates, calcium-channel blockers and beta-blockers.

The benefits of coronary bypass surgery in angina are:

- prolongation of life in multivessel disease and disease of the left coronary artery;
- disappearance of angina in 80–90% in the first year after operation; this falls to 50% free of angina by 5 years.

The mortality associated with coronary surgery is 1 to 2%, but this figure must considered against the risk of death in multivessel disease: in two-vessel disease the risk is 6% per year and in three-vessel disease 10% per year.

Myocardial infarction

Diagnosis

- *Chest pain* is in same sites as in angina but is more severe

more prolonged (over ½ hour and often several hours)
often at rest and in bed
no relief from glyceryl trinitrate.
- *Associated symptoms*:
breathlessness due to cardiac failure
sweating, nausea, vomiting
faintness and syncope due to lowered cardiac output
'angor animi' – fear of impending death
palpitations.

Sudden death – presentation

- Body may be discovered.
- Collapse and death within a few minutes with no preceding symptoms.
- Collapse and death following symptoms of 'indigestion' or 'tiredness' over past few days.
- Collapse and death within an hour or two.

Examination

No specific signs apart from a person in distress from pain and associated features of cardiac insufficiency and lowered output:

- low blood pressure
- pale cold sweating
- heart sounds 'muffled' with possible gallop rhythm
- basal lung crepitations
- pulse – tachycardia or bradycardia.

Investigation

- Electrocardiogram is mandatory in all suspected cases (Figure 15.10).
- Cardiac serum enzymes – changes only occur after 4–12 hours. They are useful confirmation of diagnosis and in prognosis.

What action should the GP consider in a patient with myocardial infarction seen at home soon after the onset?

- Relief of pain – intravenous morphine/diamorphine.
- Intravenous frusemide 20–40 mg if LV failure.
- If bradycardia (below 50) then atropine is indicated.
- If pulse is above 140 and regular, intramuscular lignocaine can be given.
- Consider referral to hospital for thrombolysis if the diagnosis is clear and the patient's condition has been stabilized by these measures.

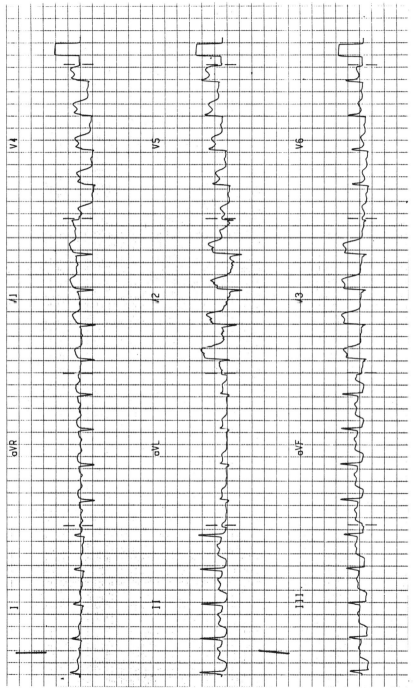

Fig. 15.10—ECG showing changes of acute-anterior myocardial infarction

Home or hospital for MI?

- The general rule should be that patients with myocardial infarction should always be referred to hospital, primarily because of the potentially fatal and completely reversible complication of ventricular fibrillation which may occur soon after the onset.
- The other important reason for patients with an infarction to be admitted to hospital is that it allows the use of a clot-dissolving drug, such as streptokinase which reduces the early mortality of myocardial infarction by 20–25%.
- However, there may be some circumstances in which it would be acceptable to treat a patient with myocardial infarction at home:

    if the onset is over 24 hours old – in these circumstances the chance of ventricular fibrillation is minimal, and streptokinase has not been shown to be of value

    if there are no other serious complications such as severe heart failure, major arrhythmias, heart block or cardiogenic shock

    if the patient is elderly and would prefer to be treated at home if possible

    if the home environment is satisfactory and relatives are available, willing and capable of looking after the patient;

    if medical advice and attention is readily available if complications do occur

    if it is the patient's preference to be treated at home.

Should GPs consider giving streptokinase at home to patients with myocardial infarction?

Although this possibility is currently being mooted, there are a number of difficulties involved:

- There is the need for the GP to have an ECG machine available to make an accurate diagnosis of infarction and also to monitor any arrhythmias which may occur following administration of the drug.
- Serious arrhythmias can occur after streptokinase has been given, and their diagnosis and treatment requires some cardiological expertise from the GP.
- Cardiac arrest may sometimes occur so there is the need of a defibrillator to be available when giving the streptokinase.
- Anaphylactic shock may occur though this should respond to intravenous hydrocortisone.
- Severe haemorrhage may occur.

Factors leading to adverse prognosis in MI:

- Early prognosis
  left ventricular failure
  shock – 90% mortality
  serious tachy-arrhythmias
  ventricular tachycardia
  ventricular fibrillation
  heart block
- Late prognosis
  depends primarily on the extent of the myocardial damage, and the main clinical pointer to this is ongoing left ventricular failure

The other complications which might influence the prognosis adversely are pulmonary, cerebro-vascular or leg peripheral emboli.

Practical points

- IHD is the major cause of death in the UK and developed countries – 27% of all deaths or 5 per GP per year.
- About ½ million new cases each year in the UK or 15 per GP and more than 1 million cases under care – 40 per GP or 200 in a group of five GPs.
- Multifactorial disease – atherosclerosis affecting coronary arteries. Most factors are individual lifestyles and family traits and genetics.
- Clinical spectrum is of angina ⅓, myocardial infarctions ⅓ and chronic heart failure and other effects ⅓.
- Angina has 4 : 3 male preponderance, with a 5-year mortality rate of 20% but 40% with no or mild symptoms. Problem is, which of moderate-severe cases (30%) should be referred for angiography.
- Exercise ECG screening test is helpful in decision-making.
- 45% of patients with myocardial infarction are dead in 5 years, including sudden deaths, and 40% have moderate–severe functional disability.
- Acute myocardial infarction should be managed in hospital coronary care units (unless good reasons for home care).

CHAPTER **16**

CARDIAC FAILURE

What is it?

Failure of the heart is the end point of life. It is a truism to state that we all die from heart failure. When the heart stops so does life.

In clinical practice however a clear distinction has to be made between philosophical end-of-life heart failure and the syndrome of clinical heart failure that we are able to diagnose, to ascribe causes to and to treat in various ways.

Acute: Acute left ventricular failure results from hypertension or acute myocardial infarction, and acute right ventricular failure from pulmonary embolism or right ventricular infarction. These are sudden, dramatic and often fatal situations, but not particularly common in primary care.

Chronic: Much more frequent are the various forms of chronic heart failure. In our ageing society more persons are living longer and are being exposed to the end results of occlusive atherosclerotic disease of the coronary arteries leading to myocardial failure, to the end results of high blood pressure and pulmonary hypertension from chronic bronchitis and emphysema. When these common causes are not apparent chronic heart failure may be caused by certain rare conditions or it may be idiopathic, that is of uncertain cause that may be in effect an 'old and worn-out heart'.

In practice then, cardiac failure is a state resulting from many possible causes. We must always try to determine the cause and endeavour to correct or cure, but more often we have to be content with the less specific therapy to control the effects of heart failure.

Definition: A failure of the heart to meet the varying metabolic and oxygen needs of the body.

In haemodynamic terms, this means an increase in end-diastolic ventricular volume and pressure with a decrease in cardiac output on exercise, or in more severe cases, at rest also.

Pathophysiology of heart failure

The pathophysiology of heart failure can be regarded as based on intrinsic disease or excessive workload.

Intrinsic disease

- ischaemic heart disease – commonest cause
- cardiomyopathy (idiopathic)
- myocarditis – from whatever cause
- myocardial infiltration causing secondary cardiomyopathy:
  amyloid disease
  sarcoidosis
  haemachromatosis

Excessive workload

(1) *Increased resistance to outflow:*
   - left ventricle:
     hypertension
     aortic stenosis
     hypertrophic obstructive cardiomyopathy
   - right ventricle:
     chronic obstructive lung disease – commonest
     pulmonary fibrosis from whatever cause
     pulmonary thrombo-embolism
     idiopathic pulmonary hypertension
(2) *Increased volume overload:*
   - aortic/mitral/tricuspid valve incompetence
   - atrial and ventricular septal defects with shunting
(3) *Excessive work demands on the heart:*
   - thyrotoxicosis
   - severe anaemia
   - pregnancy
   - Paget's disease/arteriovenous fistulae

In addition to these underlying causes, heart failure may be latent until precipitated by a triggering factor:

- sudden cardiac arrhythmia or heart block;
- systemic infection;
- strenuous exertion in a damaged heart;
- superimposed acute myocarditis, e.g. viral-associated, anaemia, thyrotoxicosis, pregnancy, onset of renal failure with sodium retention;
- sudden withdrawal of maintenance treatment, e.g. diuretics.

[The term 'congestive cardiac failure' should be avoided since it means different things to different doctors: in the USA it means left ventricular failure, in the UK it is usually taken to mean right ventricular failure, while others mean a combination of left and right ventricular failure. To avoid any ambiguity of this type when talking about heart failure it is best to use the terms left ventricular failure, right ventricular failure or biventricular failure.]

Who gets it and when?

As may be expected, cardiac failure is a condition of ageing (Figure 16.1).

The numbers involved are not great in terms of actual patients but each one with cardiac failure requires up to 10 consultations annually.

Table 16.1 shows that in a year it is chronic right ventricular heart failure that is the commonest type. Cardiac arrhythmias are part of the complex and deserve to be included although most are transient though alarming.

TABLE 16.1   Annual consultation rates for cardiac failure

Disease	Persons consulting annually per 2000	per 10 000
Chronic right ventricular heart failure	12	60
Left ventricular failure	2	10
Cor pulmonale	5	25
Cardiac arrhythmias	5	25
Total	24	120

Over the past 40 years in J.F.'s practice the numbers and percentages of the various types and causes are shown in Table 16.2 and Figure 16.2.

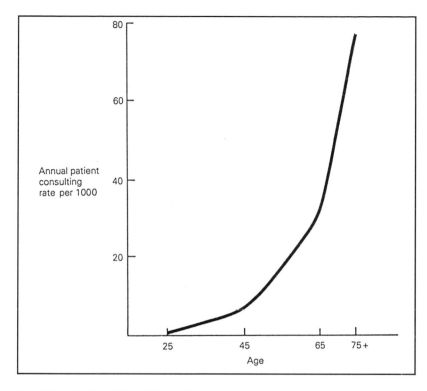

Fig. 16.1—Cardiac failure (all types) – age prevalence

TABLE 16.2   Cardiac failure: causes in a practice over 40 years

Causes of heart failure	Numbers	%
Chronic	377	68
Common: IHD	(180)	
High blood pressure	(80)	
Valvular heart disease	(57)	
Arrhythmias	(40)	
Rare: Thyroid disorders	(10)	
Constrictive pericarditis	(3)	
Subacute bacterial endocarditis	(3)	
Pulmonary embolism	(4)	
Acute LVF	75	13
Cor pulmonale	71	13
Uncertain	35	6
Total	558	100

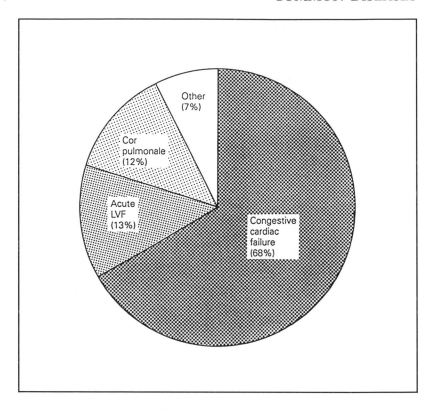

Fig. 16.2—Types of cardiac failure

How does it present?

The three *cardinal signs of left ventricular failure* are:

- breathlessness;
- a gallop rhythm on auscultating the heart;
- crepitations in the lungs.

Other signs which may be present include:

- coughing up frothy pink sputum – this is much less frequent than suggested in most text books;
- pulsus alternans – best picked up on the sphygmomanometer;
- low blood pressure (unless this is the cause of the left ventricular failure).

The three *cardinal signs of right ventricular failure* are:

- ankle and leg oedema;
- raised jugular venous pressure;
- enlarged tender congested liver.

Other signs which may be present include:

- central cyanosis (evident in the lips);
- ascites;
- sacral oedema if the patient has been recumbent for some time;
- anasarca (generalized oedema) in very severe right ventricular failure.

What happens?

A condition such as heart failure cannot be expected to have a good prognosis, but many elderly patients will continue to live with their breathlessness and oedema for a number of years. The prognosis is worse in younger patients with heart failure, unless there is a curable cause that can be corrected.

What to do

Assessment

Look for a *cause*, particularly a reversible cause, and treat if possible:

- Hypertension – treat with antihypertensives.
- Valvular heart disease – consider surgery.
- Infective endocarditis – use antibiotics.
- Thyrotoxicosis – treat with carbimazole and consider surgery if indicated when the heart failure is under control.
- Severe anaemia – careful transfusion of packed cells to avoid fluid overload and exacerbation of the heart failure.

What investigations should the GP consider doing?

- *Chest X-ray*
  Heart size – useful for prognosis.
  Degree of pulmonary congestion which indicates the severity of the left ventricular failure.
  May show possible aetiological factors: chronic obstructive lung disease or valvular heart disease, e.g. mitral stenosis.
  Atrial/ventricular septal defects: especially relevant in young patients with heart failure.
  Coarctation of the aorta – rare but eminently reversible.

- *ECG*
  Left ventricular hypertrophy – of prognostic importance in hypertensive patients.
  Evidence of previous myocardial infarction – may be cause of undiagnosed heart failure.
  May show arrhythmias which may be either the result of the heart failure or a 'trigger'.

- *Blood*
  Blood urea/creatine levels – indication of renal failure which adversely affects prognosis.
  Serum sodium/potassium levels – low serum sodium reduces the response to diuretics. Low potassium levels, as a result of diuretic treatment, encourages arrhythmias.
  Blood counts – if severe anaemia is suspected.
  Thyroid function test – if thyrotoxicosis suspected.

Management of heart failure

General measures

- No smoking – especially in chronic lung disease.
- Correct overweight.
- Reduce salt intake – no added salt at table; this will reduce the daily intake of salt to about 3 grams/day.
- Reduce intake of alcohol – excessive alcohol can cause arrhythymias and even cardiomyopathy.
- Social aid from home helps, rehousing if necessary and financial assistance.

Specific treatment

The mainstay of treatment of both left and right ventricular failure is diuretics. The place of digoxin remains controversial: it is clearly indicated if fast atrial fibrillation is present but its value in heart failure accompanied by sinus rhythm remains to be convincingly shown by controlled clinical trials in adequate numbers of patients over a reasonable length of time.

Diuretics:

- Intravenous diuretics are best in acute left ventricular failure with severe pulmonary congestion – frusemide or bumetanide are suitable drugs to inject.

- Thiazide diuretics are of little value except perhaps in maintenance treatment of mild heart failure. In addition, they may have adverse effects on blood sugar, blood urea and blood lipids. The one exception is metolazone (Metenix) which when combined with a loop diuretic such as frusemide can greatly enhance the diuretic effects.
- Loop diuretics, such as frusemide and bumetanide, are the most effective diuretics to use. The combination of frusemide and a potassium-retaining diuretic such as amiloride (Frumil) is a useful preparation to avoid long-term potassium depletion.

Angiotensin-converting enzyme inhibitors (ACEI): These drugs now play an important part in the treatment of heart failure since it has been clearly shown that they can prolong long-term survival (Norwegian Consensus Trial, 1987).

The benefits have been in treating severe left ventricular failure with enalapril (Innovace), but similar improvement has now been found with other ACE inhibitors. It is now advisable to consider their use in all patients with chronic left ventricular failure. There is one important consideration in using these drugs in patients who are already likely to be taking substantial amounts of diuretics – an excessive fall of standing blood pressure may occur when the drugs are first given. It is best, therefore, to give a *small* test dose and carefully check the response of the patient's *standing* blood pressure, in order to exclude undue sensitivity to the drug.

The place of ACE inhibitors in treating *mild* left ventricular failure and in treating right ventricular failure remains to be shown.

Other vasodilator treatment of heart failure: The basis of using vasodilators in treating heart failure is to reduce cardiac work. This can be done by reducing the 'afterload' by producing systemic arterial vasodilation, e.g. with hydralazine, or reducing the 'preload' with venodilating drugs such as nitrates (blood collects in the peripheral veins so that less returns to the heart for pumping). *

An important trial was carried out in 1986 by Cohn *et al.** showing a clear improvement in long-term survival of heart failure with a combination of hydralazine and sorbide nitrate. However, this trial has not had the same impact on the management of heart failure as the ACE inhibitor trial. We probably need more evidence of the value of this combination before accepting it as standard therapy.

* Cohn JN, Archibold DG, Franciosa JA, et al (1986) Effect of vasodilator therapy on mortality in chronic congestive heart failure. Results of a Veterans Administration Cooperative Study. N. Engl. J. Med., **314**, 1547–52.

Management of acute left ventricular failure

This is a medical emergency and needs emergency measures:

- *Diamorphine* – this is a valuable drug and its beneficial effects in left ventricular failure include:
  reduction of systolic pressure and heart rate
  depression of sensitivity of respiratory centre thus reducing feeling of dyspnoea
  allays anxiety.

NB – diamorphine should be used in minimal dosage if chronic obstructive lung disease is present, and used cautiously in the elderly.

- *Diuretics* – these drugs are the mainstay of treatment of acute left ventricular failure as well as chronic left ventricular failure. Intravenous frusemide has an important venodilator action 'offloading' the heart, as well as its main diuretic action. Bumetanide can also be used.
- *Aminophylline* i.v. – this drug has been used traditionally in acute left ventricular failure for a long time and is still a valuable drug in this condition. However, it can cause arrhythmias, and care should be taken that the patient is not already on an oral theophylline drug which may enhance its toxicity.
- *Vasodilators* – drugs such as glyceryl trinitrate or a capsule of nifedipine are always worth trying to 'offload' the heart.
- *Oxygen* – in full dosage is very important, provided that the patient does not have associated chronic airway disease, when the oxygen concentration should be reduced to no more than 28%.

Practical points

- Although we all die from failure of the heart there are definitive clinical conditions of acute and chronic cardiac failure.
- In a practice of 2000 patients 24 will consult for cardiac failure in a year.
- Almost three quarters are caused by ischaemic heart disease, high blood pressure, and pulmonary disease.
- As may be expected, cardiac failure is a condition associated with ageing.
- Assessment by the GP should include looking for a correctable cause and investigations should include chest X-ray, ECG and blood tests.
- Management must involve general self-help measures by patient and medication with diuretics and possibly ACEI and vasodilator preparations.
- Acute left ventricular failure is a medical emergency requiring urgent care at home or hospital.

CHAPTER **17**

VARICOSE VEINS

What are they?

Varicose veins are prominent veins in the lower limbs that probably affect as many as two out of three adults in some developed Western societies.

The causes are uncertain. In many there are genetic predispositions, but the trigger factor is likely to be damage to venous valves following deep vein thrombosis (silent) or trauma. They cause various symptoms. The most prominent are dislike of their cosmetic appearance and aching after standing. They are associated with complications of chronic venous insufficiency of the lower one-third of the legs with possible eczema, subcutaneous oedema and fibrosis and ulceration.

A number of treatments are possible. Long-term results of all are less than satisfactory.

Among other causal factors blamed have been overweight, type of work (standing), diet (insufficient roughage), lack of exercise, smoking, pregnancy and a family history. All may be factors in causation, but the two most definite ones proven so far have been age – the prevalence increases with every decade – and the extent of social development – varicose veins are rare in rural under-developed societies.

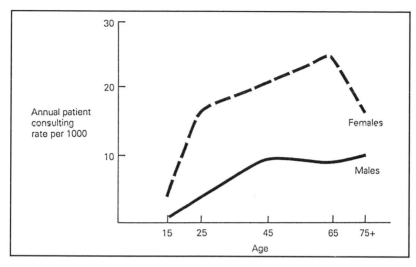

Fig. 17.1—Varicose veins – age prevalence (RCGP/OPCS, 1986)

Who gets them and when?

Although the prevalence of varicose veins in the community is high, in two-thirds of adult women and one-half of men, the actual numbers of patients consulting in a year are low, 27 in a practice of 2000 and this includes complications.

Figure 17.1 shows that of those consulting the rates in women are twice those in men and the rates increase with age.

It is likely that most persons accept them and do not seek advice.

How do they present?

The reasons for consultation in order of frequency are:

- cosmetic appearance
- aching legs
- complications such as skin changes with discolouration and thickening, eczema, ulceration and superficial or deep venous thrombosis.

What happens?

In the majority once veins have appeared they persist without complications (Figure 17.2).

- Varicose eczema occurs in 15%.
- Fibrotic thickening and induration of lower third of leg in 10%.
- Varicose ulceration in 3%.

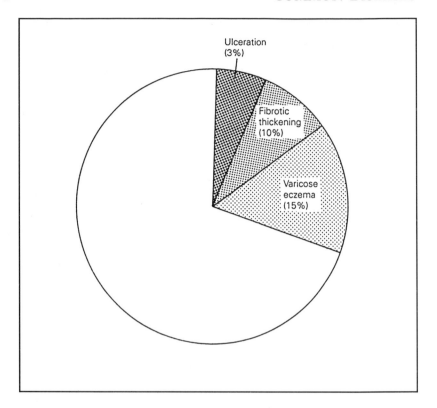

Fig. 17.2—Varicose veins – complications

What to do

The key issue in assessment in persons with varicose veins is to decide who needs treatment and what treatment?

The indications for treatment in most cases are the patient's choice and concern with the appearance of the legs and minor symptoms.

The choice in advising treatment will be:

- none at present, but reassurance
- elastic supportive stockings
- injection-compression
- surgical removal (stripping) and ligation of perforating veins.

Whatever treatment is given the results become increasingly poor with time. With injection-compression after 5 years about one-half need further treatment. With surgery after 5 years about one-quarter need further treatment.

Practical points

- Varicose veins are common in developed societies (2 out of 3 adults having some) but rare in rural developing societies.
- Most persons do not seek medical advice.
- In a practice of 2000 only 27 will consult in a year for varicose veins and complications.
- Eczema occurs in 15%, fibrotic induraton in 10% and *ulceration* in 3%.
- Supportive stockings relieve symptoms; results of injection-compression (50% recur) and surgery (25% recur) are poor.

CHAPTER **18**

ANAEMIA

What is it?

'Anaemia' is not a specific condition but a sign of some underlying disorder such as:

- unsuspected continuing blood loss usually from gastro-intestinal tract or uterus
- defective blood production due to deficiency of essential factors such as vitamin B12, folic acid, or iron from inadequate intake or malabsorption
- excessive blood destruction from haemolysis
- bone marrow dysfunction
- others associated with systemic diseases such as kidney and liver failure, cancers and rheumatoid disease.

In general practice the majority of anaemias are iron-deficiency types associated with excessive and often unsuspected blood loss.

Who gets it and when?

There is a considerable difference between the number of patients who consult and are diagnosed as anaemic and those undiagnosed in the community.

Taking less than 12g per 100ml of haemoglobin as the criterion for anaemia, the annual patient consulting rate for anaemia is around 20 in a practice of 2000.

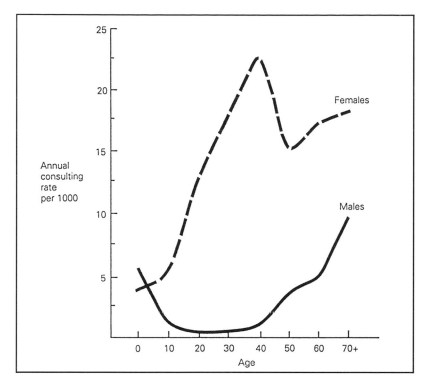

Fig. 18.1—Anaemia – clinical incidence (consulting rates)

In a screening exercise of adults in J.F.'s practice a point prevalence rate of 80 per 2000 was found.

Figure 18.1 shows:

- High prevalence of anaemia in women during reproductive age period 20–50 – due to excessive blood loss during menstruation or deficient iron intake.
- Rising prevalence in both sexes from age 50 onwards due to hidden continuing blood loss from various gastro-intestinal diseases such as oesophagitis, bowel cancers and piles; inadequate diets; side-effects from drugs; inefficient bone marrow activity.
- In infancy haemoglobin levels tend to be low in some children, a mixture of 'physiological' anaemia and iron-deficient diet. Here the prevalence is higher in males.

The types of anaemia in practice are:

• iron deficiency	85%
• megaloblastic	10%
• others	5%

How do they present?

Anaemia is silent and often a surprise finding. There are no characteristic clinical features.

Pallor, listlessness, tiredness, depression, sore tongue, breathlessness and dysphagia may be symptoms and signs of anaemia but they occur often when there is no anaemia in patients with depression and other disorders.

The clinical approach must be for a high degree of awareness of the possibility of anaemia in women (20–50 years), in the elderly and in infants.

What happens?

The natural history and outcome in anaemia must be that of the underlying cause, but in the most frequent group, that in women aged 20–50, unless regular and constant supervision is undertaken and the iron deficiency corrected, there will be recurrence of the anaemia. Anaemia was evident in one-third of such defaulters followed-up (J.F.).

What to do?

If an accurate diagnosis of anaemia is to be made and underlying causes discovered, the physician must have access to modern and reliable diagnostic investigations. A purely clinical diagnosis of 'anaemia' is dangerous and unreliable and no such diagnostic label should ever be attached without confirmation by further investigations.

In the field of primary care where the diagnosis of anaemia will follow a clinical 'alert', many excessive investigations will be undertaken in which the results will be normal. Therefore it is necessary to arrive at some simple minimal tests which can serve as a reliable initial screen, to pick up anaemia and to serve as a guide to the type of anaemia and to any further investigations.

As a minimum the following tests are necessary: haemoglobin level, packed cell volume per cent, mean cell haemoglobin concentration per cent and an examination of the smear showing the appearance of the blood cells.

If anaemia is found, then further haematological and other investigations may be required, such as radiology of the chest and gastro-intestinal tract, and occult blood in stools.

Physical examination should concentrate on the gastro-intestinal tract and the female genital tract to discover any obvious causes of bleeding.

It is essential that a definite diagnosis of exact type of megaloblastic anaemia can be made before any vitamin B12 or folic acid is given as treatment. Massive blind blunderbuss therapy will add to the difficulties and confusion in diagnosis.

Good management of anaemia comprises:

- accurate diagnosis
- definitive treatment
- long-term follow-up.

The need for accurate diagnosis has been stressed already and it must consist of confirmatory blood tests, clinical examination and further investigations, where necessary.

Definitive treatment will depend on the diagnosis of the cause. Any discovered primary condition, such as uterine fibroids and other gynaecological abnormalities, bleeding piles, peptic ulcers, deficient diet, etc. must be corrected.

The most common type of anaemia is an *iron deficiency anaemia* from excessive blood loss and a deficient iron intake. It is useless giving iron without taking steps to control excessive blood loss.

Iron is best given by mouth as an additional supplement of the diet. Provided that the dose of iron is adequate and providing that the patient does not suffer from a malabsorption syndrome, oral iron will produce as rapid a rise as parenteral intramuscular or intravenous therapy.

The type of oral iron preparation is probably not important except in those who cannot tolerate simple preparations such as ferrous sulphate or gluconate. In these, longer acting, slow-release preparations may be tolerated better.

Combined preparations of iron with other haematinics are not recommended except in pregnancy where a combination of iron and folic acid may be used.

Whatever preparation is used and tolerated, it is essential that the patient understands that iron supplement intake must be continued until excessive blood loss such as menorrhagia ceases. The commonest cause of recurrent and refractory anaemia is the discontinuation of iron supplements by the patient.

Megaloblastic anaemia is uncommon. The prevalence is probably around 1–2 per 1000, so that a practice with 2000 persons will have some 3–4 patients needing long-term therapy. Pernicious anaemia caused by lack of an intrinsic factor which leads to defective absorption of vitamin B12, is the most frequent type of megaloblastic anaemia in practice.

Patients with pernicious anaemia, once stabilized, need an injection of hydroxocobalamin, 1000 micrograms every 2–3 months for the rest of their lives. A blood check of haemoglobin level should be done once or twice a year.

Follow-up: All patients with anaemia should be followed up and their haemoglobin levels checked periodically to ensure that their anaemia remains controlled.

A special type is the patient who has had gastric surgery. These patients should have their haemoglobin levels checked annually. Anaemia is frequent after gastrectomy (up to a 50% risk) and not infrequent after vagotomy and drainage.

Another especially vulnerable type is the old person living alone on a poor diet. Here, as well as treating the anaemia, social measures must be taken to correct the underlying isolation and self-neglect.

Practical points

- Anaemia is a common condition often missed and untreated.
- Annual incidence of new cases is 20 per 2000 population.
- It is possible that there are four times as many undiagnosed persons with anaemia (albeit slight) in the community.
- 85% are iron deficiency anaemias, 10% megaloblastic anaemias and 5% are other varieties.
- The likely causes of iron deficiency anaemia are excessive menstrual bleeding, blood loss from gastro-intestinal tract as in piles, hiatus hernia/oesophagitis, peptic ulcers and neoplasms; and from deficient diets.
- Iron replacement may correct the situation temporarily but anaemia will recur if the primary causal condition is not corrected.
- Long-term management supervision of all types of anaemia is necessary as well as screening of possible at-risk groups such as post-gastrectomy cases.

SECTION IV

GASTRO-INTESTINAL DISEASES

CHAPTER 19

GASTRO-INTESTINAL DISEASES – THE CLINICAL SPECTRUM

The clinical spectrum of gastro-intestinal diseases ranges from minor infections with acute vomiting and diarrhoea, which are wellnigh endemic; functional dyspeptic symptoms and vague undiagnosed abdominal pains through specific conditions such as peptic ulcers and chronic intestinal inflammatory disorders; to life-threatening acute abdominal emergencies and cancers.

It is important to have a proper perspective of the rates of frequency of these various conditions.

Patient consulting rates

The importance of gastro-intestinal diseases is evident from the fact that one-quarter of all persons who consulted in the Third National Morbidity Study (18% of the population) did so for these disorders.

Table 19.1 shows the expected numbers of persons consulting in a year, in a practice of 2000 and in a group of 10 000.

TABLE 19.1   Annual patient consulting rates

Condition	per 2000	per 10 000
Dental and mouth disorders	34	170
Acute gastro-intestinal infections	68	340
Oesophageal disorders and hiatus hernia	14	70
Peptic ulcers	12	60
(duodenal)	(9)	(45)
(gastric)	(3)	(15)
Functional disorders of stomach	32	160
Appendicitis and acute abdomen	6	30
Hernia	10	50
(inguinal)	(6)	
(femoral)	(2)	
(other)	(2)	
Intestinal–chronic inflammatory	2	10
Diverticular disease	4	20
Irritable bowel syndrome	24	120
Rectal and anal	8	40
Haemorrhoids	16	80
Constipation	18	90
Gall bladder, liver, pancreas	8	40
Cancers	4	20
Symptoms – dyspepsia	44	220
Symptoms – abdominal pain	60	300

Note that the most prevalent groups were for the less specific conditions such as presumed acute gastro-intestinal infections, undiagnosed abdominal pain, dyspeptic symptoms, what is termed 'functional disorders of the stomach', and the uncertain 'irritable bowel syndrome'.

Note also the relatively small numbers of life-threatening conditions such as cancer and acute abdominal emergencies.

The physician must accept that two-thirds are these vague conditions of indefinite nature that have to be managed nevertheless.

Consultation rates

With an annual consultation rate of 3.4 (or 3400 per 1000) consultations per person, consultations for gastro-intestinal disorders were 277 per 1000 or 8% of all consultations.

Sickness and invalidity

Six per cent of all days and spells of sickness and invalidity are due to gastro-intestinal disorders.

Hospital in-patient data

Most admissions are for surgical procedures. Overall 8% of all hospital admissions are for gastro-intestinal disorders.

Causes of death

11% of deaths are caused by gastro-intestinal diseases (Table 19.2).

TABLE 19.2   Deaths from gastro-intestinal disease

Cause	Deaths	%
Cancers	50 000	71
Peptic ulcers	5 000	7
Liver, gall bladder, pancreas	5 000	7
Acute abdomen	4 000	6
Others	6 000	9
Total deaths from gastro-intestinal disease	70 000	
Total deaths	(600 000)	

CHAPTER **20**

ACUTE
GASTROENTERITIS

Just as acute respiratory infections are the most common type of respiratory disease in the community, so acute gastroenteritis is the most frequent disorder of gastro-intestinal diseases. It accounts for one-fifth of all persons consulting for gastro-intestinal diseases.

Having noted the high prevalence of gastroenteritis it has to be acknowledged that we scarcely know what this common condition is. Its symptomatology is well recognized but its causes less so.

Two forms may be recognized epidemiologically, the endemic and the epidemic types.

The endemic type of acute gastroenteritis is present constantly in the community. Every day of every week the family physician will be consulted by persons with acute vomiting and/or diarrhoea. There may be other cases in the household but quite often such episodes occur singly. These are the more frequent type.

The epidemic type of acute gastroenteritis has a more explosive, extensive and dramatic picture – sudden onset, numbers of cases occurring simultaneously. This epidemic type is less frequent and often is caused by a single common food or water source of infection. It tends to occur more in closed communities such as schools, camps, canteens (or restaurants), or from a water source affecting a fairly well-defined geographical area.

216

Visitors to other lands often experience a bout of acute gastro-enteritis that is often given fanciful names such as 'gyppy tummy' or 'Montezuma's revenge'. It is as though visitors' gastro-intestinal tracts are unfamiliar with local strains of common organisms and that time is necessary for immunity to develop.

The significance of acute gastroenteritis differs with the age of the victim and the social class. The condition is potentially more serious and dangerous in young children and in lower social groups.

Even if every case of acute gastroenteritis were to be investigated for possible pathogenic organisms, such organisms would be detected in less than 10% of all attacks. The rate will be higher in exceptional epidemics caused by food or water-borne organisms.

The fact that in so many attacks no pathogenic organisms are detected means either that the attacks of acute gastroenteritis are caused by organisms which are not detectable or that the conditions are not true infections.

The alternative explanation may be that our present diagnostic methods are inadequate for isolation.

It may be that many attacks of gastroenteritis are caused by viruses but this cannot be accepted as a fact until effective methods are developed to isolate the causal organisms and subject them to Koch's postulates.

The organisms that may be isolated are:

- Bacterial:
  Escherichia coli
  Dysentery caused by *Shigella sonnei*
  Salmonella infections of various types
  Staphylococcal food poisoning
  Clostridial food poisoning
  Cholera
  Campylobacter.
- Protozoal:
  Giardia lamblia
  Entamoeba histolytica.

There are other situations which may present as 'acute gastro-enteritis' (see pages 244–252) and which have to be considered in diagnosis.

Who gets it when?

Figure 20.1 shows that acute gastroenteritis is frequent in infancy and childhood, but after the first decade the annual prevalence is

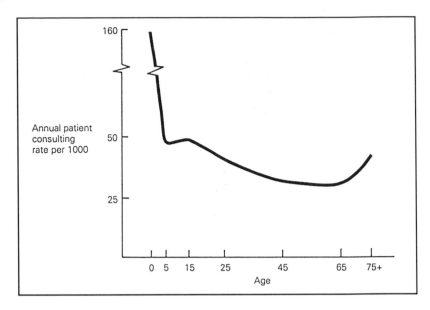

Fig 20.1—Acute gastroenteritis – annual patient consulting rates

almost constant. The condition is equally frequent in males and in females.

In a practice of 2000, 68 persons consult in a year for acute gastroenteritis (page 214) but the actual numbers of cases in the community are many times greater, being self-managed.

How does it present?

The prominent presenting features are vomiting and/or diarrhoea. The two may occur together or there may be vomiting without diarrhoea or diarrhoea without vomiting.

Vomiting is associated with nausea and intense malaise in adults. There are no special characteristics of the vomitus. Abdominal pain may be absent but usually there is some discomfort. There may be an epigastric ache with vomiting or griping colicky mid-abdominal pains accompanying diarrhoea.

Diarrhoea consists of frequent watery semi-formed motions. There may be mucus present but blood is not usual. If blood is noted it may be due to a dysenteric infection or to some major non-infective condition.

The general condition may be little disturbed in a short and sharp attack. Rarely, in infants, in debilitated persons and in severe

attacks there may be profound disturbance, collapse and even
death.

Dehydration is a potential danger in infants when vomiting and
diarrhoea are frequent and profuse and when prolonged for more
than 24 hours. Dehydration is unusual in adults unless the attack
is severe and persistent.

What happens?

The usual course of a non-specific attack is for the symptoms to
clear spontaneously over 2 or 3 days. Where the condition persists
then a reassessment of cause and management are necessary.

What to do?

Assessment

In most attacks of 'D and V' there is no need for specific therapy
or for anxiety on the part of the physician. With suitable advice
on adequate fluid consumption and avoidance of solid food,
dehydration should not occur. Special care and supervision are
necessary when managing infants and elderly persons.

Questions that arise when managing persons with 'D and V' are:

- Are there other cases in the home or in the area?
- May there be a common cause such as food poisoning or water
  contamination?
- Does the patient work in a food trade and is further transmission
  of infection possible?
- Has the patient been travelling abroad recently?

Apart from common acute infections vomiting and/or diarrhoea
may occur as presenting features in the following major diseases:

- acute appendicitis
- diverticulitis
- cancer of the large gut
- colitis
- diabetes
- mesenteric thrombosis
- intussusception
- food sensitivities (or enzyme disorders)
- metabolic disorders, as in diabetes, thyrotoxicosis and Addison's
  disease
- excessive alcohol

- iatrogenic effects from overdosage with laxatives
- meningitis.

Careful consideration must be given to these possible causes in any case that departs from the normal course.

Most attacks settle quickly and investigations are not necessary as a routine.

If symptoms are not clearing after a few days or if there are unusual clinical features then alternative diagnoses must be considered.

The main points in management are:

(1) Since the causes of the majority of attacks are uncertain and since the course usually is towards a natural and spontaneous recovery in 2–3 days, specific treatment is unnecessary.

(2) General advice includes: no solid food for 1–2 days and plentiful clear fluids. For the short sharp attack the type of fluid is unimportant.

(3) There is no need for non-specific medication.

(4) There are few indications for antibiotics. Certainly they should not be given blindly without a specific pathogen having been isolated. There is no evidence that antibiotics or chemotherapy are helpful in dysentery infections or even in most salmonella infections. Metronidazole is a specific remedy for *Giardia lamblia*. Chloramphenicol or cotrimoxazole may be indicated in typhoid fever. Metronidazole or emetine are necessary in amoebic dysentery.

(5) The patient and/or family must be informed of the likely course towards natural improvement within 48–72 hours. If such improvement does not occur or there is anxiety over the condition of the patient then urgent reassessment is necessary by the physician.

(6) Infancy – more precise instructions are necessary for parents. The essence of management is maintenance of adequate fluid intake:

- no solids or milk until vomiting stops
- breast feeding can continue
- give clear fluids – water, 'flat' lemonade or squash – a little and often
- give fluids even if child vomits
- after 24–48 hours, restart on diluted milk
- glucose-electrolyte preparations (Dioralyte) can be used as alternative to 'clear fluids'.

If no improvement with 24–48 hours or if signs of dehydration – then admit to hospital.

Practical points

- Acute gastroenteritis is the most prevalent gastro-intestinal disorder.
- It affects all persons at all ages in all countries.
- Endemic ('There's a lot of it around') and epidemic varieties occur, the former the more frequent.
- Many possible causes of the common symptoms of diarrhoea and vomiting (D and V) but, except in special situations, it is unnecessary to seek the cause.
- The special situations in which efforts should be made to isolate the causal organism are:
  local epidemics possibly due to food poisoning
  recent arrivals from overseas.
- Maximal prevalence in infancy.
- Usually short sharp attack without complications.
- May be dangerous from dehydration in infants, elderly and those with other diseases.
- No specific anti-bacterial therapy is necessary but it is important to maintain fluid and electrolyte balance.

CHAPTER 21

FUNCTIONAL DISORDERS OF GI TRACT

What are they?

Second only to acute 'D and V' (gastroenteritis) are a vague group of symptomatic disorders of function of the gastro-intestinal tract. They make up one-quarter of the total of persons consulting for gastro-intestinal diseases in primary care. In a practice of 2000 persons, this means 178 persons in a year.

Collected together these conditions produce symptoms from the top to the bottom of the GI tract – from flatulence, heartburn and nausea, through abdominal pains, to constipation and diarrhoea.

Although they are classified together, their causation, nature and course are far from being clearly understood.

Three symptom-complexes can be distinguished (Table 21.1), but there may be considerable overlap. There is a group with symptoms related to the upper GI tract: heartburn, nausea, flatulence and 'disordered function of the stomach'; there are those who present chiefly with abdominal pains; and those with constipation and/or diarrhoea.

TABLE 21.1   Patients consulting annually for functional GI disorders

Diagnosis	Annual persons consulting	
	per 2000	per 10 000
Functional disorders of stomach	32	160
Irritable bowel syndrome	24	120
Constipation	18	90
'Dyspepsia'	44	220
'Abdominal pain'	60	300

Causes

With such a collection of symptoms it is not surprising that there are many suggestions as to possible causes.

However, it is important to consider these functional diagnostic labels as ones of exclusion, only after possible treatable and serious organic diseases have been searched for.

All these symptoms may be early symptoms of various neoplasms of the GI tract, hiatus hernia, peptic ulcers, gall bladder, liver or pancreatic diseases, Crohn's disease, diverticulosis and other more rare conditions.

Having considered and excluded these diseases, there are left a large number of persons with these symptom complexes, outnumbering peptic ulcers by 4 : 1, outnumbering gall bladder, liver and pancreatic diseases by 12 : 1, and outnumbering cancers of the GI tract by 50 : 1. These functional disorders are some of the most common, persistent and recurrent conditions in developed societies.

The following have been suggested as possible causes, but there is no definite proof for any of them:

- Emotional and psychosomatic factors, often with a personality diathesis and a family history of similar problems.
- Diet factors, such as lack of roughage, or too much roughage, or sensitivity to foods such as sugar, milk, coffee, tea, alcohol, etc.
- Stresses and strains of modern life, a useful and non-provable collection of factors.
- Iatrogenic factors, such as too many laxatives or too much consumption of substances such as aspirin and codeine derivatives.
- Aftermaths of past gastro-intestinal infections.

Whatever the true causes may be, the implications for management must be that we are unsure and that persons suffering from these conditions must be managed as individuals with their own special problems.

Who gets them and when?

Figures 21.1–21.3 show the age prevalence rates for the three groups of conditions. The patterns are different.

Abdominal pains are twice as frequent in women as in men. The peak age prevalence is in the young and middle-aged with a decline after 60 (Figure 21.1). This prevalence pattern is similar to other conditions such as duodenal ulcers, migraine, and anxiety-depression which all have possible psychosomatic aetiologies.

Constipation (Figure 21.2) has a different age prevalence curve, being most frequent in the young and the old. Here too there is a 2 : 1 female predominance.

The group of **symptoms related to the upper GI tract** (Figure 21.3) shows yet another different age prevalence pattern. The frequency increases with age, being most likely in the elderly. Here the conditions are distributed equally in males and in females. This curve is characteristic of disorders associated with ageing and degenerative processes, such as rheumatism, coronary artery disease and high blood pressure, chronic bronchitis, cancer and strokes (see Chapter 47).

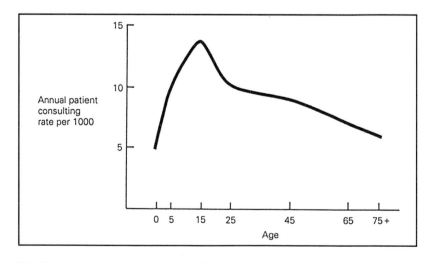

Fig. 21.1—Abdominal pain – age prevalence

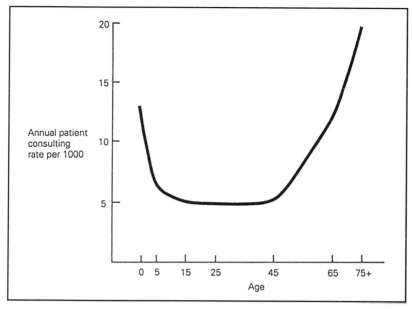

Fig. 21.2—Constipation and diarrhoea – age prevalence

Clinical syndromes

There are no specific clear-cut symptoms and signs and observations must be general.

Recurrent abdominal pain in children

This is common in the 4–8 year age group. Usually occurring in the morning prior to going to school or in association with some other stressful situation for the child. The pain is referred by the child to the umbilicus. Pain may be accompanied by vomiting, pallor or headache. Symptoms tend to cease after 7–8 years of age, but some children may grow up into adults who are prone to suffer from recurrent abdominal pains or headaches.

Irritable bowel syndrome

This tends to affect women more than men and in the 30–60 age period. The symptoms are recurrent or constant aching pain in the left abdomen, but it can occur anywhere in the abdomen. There may be attacks of colicky pains. Pain may occasionally be sited in left upper quadrant and referred to left chest and arm. Abdominal distension is a complaint.

Constipation is usual, but morning diarrhoea may affect some victims, either alone or alternating with constipation.

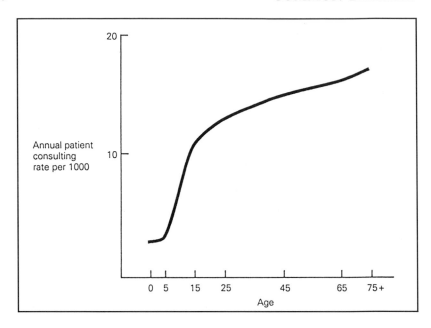

Fig. 21.3—Disordered function of the stomach – age prevalence

The tendency is for symptoms to cease naturally in time. There are no associations with more serious organic diseases such as cancer or diverticulosis.

The irritable bowel can be managed on the following lines:

- After assessment and investigation, the patient should be reassured with an explanation of the condition and its course.
- It is worth trying the effects of a high-roughage bran diet.
- Constipation should be relieved by the above diet but until then bowel bulk-increasing preparations or senna preparations can be used.
- Morning diarrhoea and abdominal pains respond well to codeine phosphate (15–30 mg) at night and repeated during the day as necessary.

Non-ulcer dyspepsia

This title includes the many and various forms of upper GI symptoms, such as heartburn, flatulence, nausea and upper abdominal discomfort.

Apart from describing the symptoms there are no definable syndromes. Since these symptoms are ones of exclusion, they are not related to peptic ulcers, gall bladder, liver or pancreatic diseases.

Constipation

Constipation is common in modern developed societies. The true frequency is uncertain but some 10% of Western society populations take laxatives regularly. Constipation is rare in rural and developing communities.

The current explanation is over-purified and low-roughage foods in developed countries.

It is difficult to allocate specific symptoms to constipation apart from general discomfort and possibly anal complications such as fissures and haemorrhoids.

The pathophysiology of constipation still remains unclear. There may be an organic disturbance of the nerve plexus in the colon in some longstanding cases. The histological changes found in these cases used to be thought to be due to chronic laxative abuse, but this view is now being questioned and it is possible that underlying organic disease of the myoneural plexuses in the colonic wall may be a contributory factor in causing the constipation.

Oesophagus

Reflux oesophagitis – may lead to chemical damage to oesophagus from regurgitated acid.

Pathophysiology

Incompetence of lower oesophageal sphincter, abnormal peristalsis leading to poor clearance of acid from oesophagus.

Symptoms:

- heartburn
- diffuse dull oesophageal pain
- oesophageal 'colic' – severe deep-seated gripping pain in the centre of the chest sometimes radiating through to the back/throat/epigastrium/arms
- dysphagia in the absence of organic stricture
- angina-like pain in the presence of normal coronary arteries. 20% of patients admitted to hospital with chest pain have an oesophageal cause for the pain. Tests which may help to differentiate angina from oesophageal pain include:
  exercise ECG
  acid perfusion into the oesophagus to see if the pain is   reproduced

barium swallow X-ray
endoscopy
oesophageal pH and pressure monitoring.

Complications of chronic gastro-oesophageal regurgitation:

oesophageal stricture
oesophageal ulceration
• Barrett's oesophagus – replacement of the normal squamous
 epithelium at the lower end of the oesophagus by metaplastic
 columnar epithelium – may lead to the development of oesophageal
 cancer
• anaemia – due to blood loss from oesophageal ulceration.

Management of heartburn due to gastro-oesophageal reflux:

Affects most people at some time. 60% of the population have or
have had some form of dyspepsia and in 70% of these it is
heartburn.

• Reduce obesity.
• Dietary change – avoid fat, chocolate, coffee, spices and citrus
 juices.
• Stop smoking – smoking has an adverse effect on both the
 oesophageal mucosa and the sphincter.
• Reduce alcohol intake.
• Drugs – stop any NSAIDs if possible.
• Try antacids and alginate preparations, e.g. Gaviscon.
• H_2-blockers – if no improvement: cimetidine (Tagamet),
 ranitidine (Zantac).
• Drugs which improve oesophageal motility may help, e.g.
 metoclopramide (Maxolon).

If the heartburn remains resistant, the other measures which can
be considered include:

• reconsider the diagnosis
• endoscopy and oesophageal pH measuring
• omeprazole (Losec) 4 at night for 4 weeks – if effective maintain
 treatment with conventional H_2-blockers
• surgery.

Stomach

50% of dyspeptic symptoms are associated with no evidence of
peptic ulceration or inflammation in the upper intestine. This
non-ulcer dyspepsia is probably caused by a disturbed gastric
motility pattern, especially delayed gastric emptying:

- post-prandial nausea/vomiting
- upper abdominal discomfort
- feeling of fullness after meals
- bloating and distension
- flatulence (belching)
- excessive 'rumbling' may occur.

Management

- Diet – small, frequent meals which help to avoid abdominal distension.
- Metoclopramide (Maxolon) or cisapride (Prepulsid – much more expensive) may improve gastric motility.
- Erythromycin – an interesting new approach to improving gastric motility, especially gastric emptying. The long-term effects of this treatment have not yet been assessed.

Assessment

Since these conditions of 'functional disorder' are diagnoses of exclusion, consideration must be given to other possibilities before making the diagnosis.

Not every case with flatulence, heartburn, nausea, abdominal pains or constipation has to be investigated in detail and depth but in every case alternative differential diagnoses must be considered.

In order of importance:

- GI neoplasms
- peptic ulcers
- gall bladder, liver and pancreatic diseases

have to be considered and if indicated appropriate investigations carried out to exclude them.

As well as consideration being given to possible alternative specific conditions, careful assessment must be given to the patient, as an individual with her (or his) personality, personal, family and work situations and any underlying problems or anxieties, or psychiatric disorders noted and managed where necessary.

What happens?

With a collection of different conditions no overall predictions are possible:

- Some children with recurrent abdominal pains continue to suffer as adults and may be prone to migraine-type headaches.

- Irritable bowel syndrome tends to be a condition of young and middle-aged adults and symptoms become less in elderly.
- Constipation persists unless considerable changes are made to a more bulky diet.
- Oesophageal dyspepsia is likely to persist and complications such as anaemia and oesophageal stricture are not uncommon.
- Gastric symptoms are often the result of excessive smoking, alcohol and lifestyles, and may be relieved with patient collaboration.

Practical points

- Functional GI symptoms are common: 178 patients consulting annually per 2000 population.
- Nature and causes are uncertain and probably include a mixture of personal susceptibilities, lifestyles, diet and side-effects of medication.
- Definable syndromes include recurrent abdominal pain in children, irritable bowel syndrome, gastro-oesophageal disorders and constipation.
- Course and outcome depend on possible causal factors but there is a general tendency to improvement with age.
- Symptoms may be relieved with various medications.

CHAPTER 22

PEPTIC ULCERS

What are they?

There are many ways of defining peptic ulcers – on clinical, endoscopic, radiological and pathological criteria.

Peptic ulcers are symptom-complexes in which the diagnosis of duodenal or gastric ulcer is confirmed by endoscopic and radiological appearances and in a few at surgery or autopsy through pathological appearances.

The pathology of gastric or duodenal ulcers is that they are ulcerations of the mucosa and underlying structures, usually of the first part of duodenum or the lesser curve of the stomach. They often occur singly, but they may be multiple, and whilst gastric and duodenal ulcers tend to be separate and distinct disorders, the two may coexist.

The true causes of peptic ulcers are not known, although numerous theories exist. Whilst we are aware of many associated factors such as hyper-acidity, blood groups, family susceptibility, stress of life and others, there is no understanding of why peptic ulcers occur.

Helicobacter pylori: This is an organism which is often found in the mucous layers of the gastric mucosa, and is associated with histological gastritis and postulated to be a cause of peptic ulceration. The frequency of its presence increases with age – it occurs in 20% of 20-year-olds and 60% of 60-year-olds. It is almost invariably present in patients with duodenal ulcer, and its eradication reduces the rate of relapse after treatment. *Helicobacter pylori* is most effectively found by biopsy of the antral mucosa. Bismuth preparations, e.g. DeNol, used in the treatment of peptic ulcer can inhibit the growth of the organism, but its elimination is best achieved by a one week's course of metronidazole 400 mg t.d.s. and amoxycillin 250 mg t.d.s.

Clinically, the characteristic features are epigastric pain, relieved by food and alkalis, and a certain periodicity related to meals, time of day and stress.

Endoscopy is the most reliable method of diagnosing gastric or duodenal ulcer, and offers the additional facility of obtaining a biopsy, an essential requirement if there is any possibility of the gastric ulcer being malignant. Some gastroenterologists consider that all *gastric* ulcers should be confirmed on endoscopy and a biopsy taken because of their propensity for malignancy.

Radiology (double-contrast barium meal) has been a traditional investigation for peptic ulcer, but there is often difficulty in distinguishing scarring due to old duodenal ulceration from acute ulceration. Superficial ulceration may also be missed.

Gastric or duodenal ulcers, then, are collections of recognized and defined symptoms which when supported by a positive radiological and/or endoscopic report lead to the firm diagnosis of peptic ulcer. Note that asymptomatic ulceration can occur in elderly persons taking non-steroidal anti-inflammatory drugs (NSAIDs).

Who gets them and when?

Peptic ulcers have become less prevalent over the past 40 years in J.F.'s practice. From the 1950s through to the 1970s the *annual incidence* of *new cases* (confirmed radiologically) was at a rate of 4–5 per 1000. Over the past 12 years (1980–1992) the rate has diminished to 2–3 per 1000.

The *annual patient consulting rate* per 2000 is 12, and 60 per 10 000.

As will be seen (on page 236) there is a tendency in time for persons with diagnosed peptic ulcers to cease suffering symptoms. It means that in a practice of 2000 there may be up to 100 persons with present or past history of peptic ulcers.

Duodenal ulcers are more frequent than gastric ulcers (4:1).

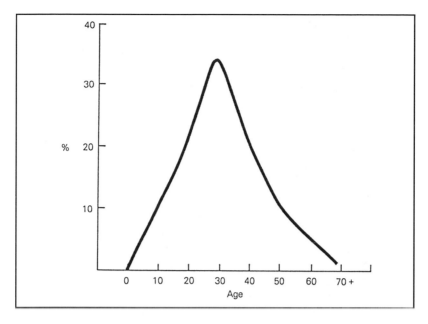

Fig. 22.1—Duodenal ulcers – peak onset at ages 20–40

The *ages at first diagnosis* differ. Duodenal ulcers on diagnosis are most likely at ages 20–40; gastric ulcers later, at ages 40–60, (Figures 22.1 and 22.2)

The *age prevalence* (persons consulting) of peptic ulcers (Figures 22.3 and 22.4) shows different patterns in the two types:

- *duodenal ulcers* (males most frequent) are seen most often at 30–50
- *gastric ulcers* (equal frequency in the two sexes) – prevalence increases with age.

Duodenal ulcers appear to be more prevalent than expected in persons with –

- chronic bronchitis
- ischaemic heart disease
- chronic renal disease.

Gastric ulcers are more prevalent in persons with pulmonary tuberculosis.

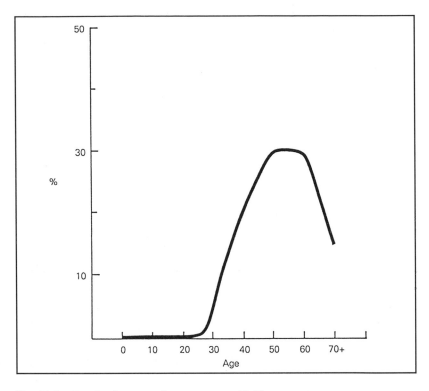

Fig. 22.2—Gastric ulcers – peak onset at ages 40–60

How do they present?

The characteristic clinical feature of peptic ulcer is the character of abdominal pain experienced.

The pain is central and epigastric. It is described as dull and gnawing. The site is often well demarcated by the patient discretely pointing with a finger rather than placing his whole hand across the upper abdomen. The pain may extend to the back or up the chest pre-sternally.

Although the pain of duodenal ulcer is described characteristically as occurring before meals and that of gastric ulcer after meals, there is considerable overlap; therefore the timing of the pain is not reliable as a guide to the type of ulcer. A more helpful symptom is the occurrence of nocturnal pain in duodenal ulcer – this is rare in gastric ulcer.

Relief of the pain is obtained by eating, drinking milk or taking alkaline preparations.

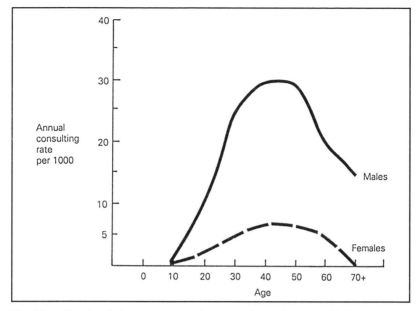

Fig. 22.3—Duodenal ulcers, more prevalent in males, peak at ages 35–55

Vomiting is not a common feature of peptic ulcers, unless there is duodenal or gastric obstruction from spasm, or organic constrictive pyloric stenosis. However, some individuals find that emptying the stomach by induced vomiting will relieve pain.

Appetite remains normal in duodenal ulcers, but the patient becomes afraid to eat because of the association of pain with eating.

In gastric ulcers the appetite is often appreciably reduced quite apart from the fear of eating.

Waterbrash is a feature of duodenal ulcers and associated heartburn is the result of gastro-oesophageal acid reflux.

Periodicity is a feature of duodenal ulcers. Bouts of abdominal pain and other symptoms are characteristic, with intervening periods of complete freedom. It is difficult to find any common trigger factors, but individuals discover that certain foods or situations may start an attack.

The course may be that of a single attack of pain over a few weeks, with no subsequent troubles. A series of bouts may recur over many years, reaching a crescendo climax, and then becoming less frequent and less severe. Continuing and increasing attacks with little respite may be the pattern.

The most usual course is that of onset-peak-recovery over some 5–10 years, with eventual cessation of symptoms.

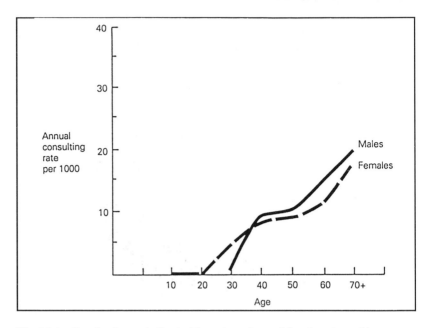

Fig. 22.4—Gastric ulcers, similar incidence in males and females, rises with age

What happens?

Peptic ulcers cause symptoms but can also cause deaths from complications such as bleeding and perforation (5000 deaths annually in the UK).

There is a natural tendency for symptoms of duodenal ulcers to remit with time, less so with gastric ulcers.

It is suggested that even without specific treatment,

- 40% heal in 4 weeks
- 60% heal in 6 weeks
- 80% heal in 8 weeks.

However, *recurrences* are frequent and in 80% symptoms recur within 12 months.

Eventually, after a period of intermittent activity for 10–15 years, symptoms tend to cease in the majority.

In the past, prior to availability of specific anti-ulcer drugs, J.F. found that in 15–20% severe symptoms required surgery by vagotomy or gastrectomy (more often with gastric ulcers).

Now the rate of surgery is much lower, but may be indicated in resistant cases where there is a possibility of pre-malignancy in gastric ulcer.

Complications may occur:

- bleeding in 10–15%
- perforation in 1–2%.

Bleeding presents as *haematemesis* or *melaena* with loose, black tarry, rancid, pungent stools or as a *sudden faint*.

A more slowly bleeding ulcer may lead to symptoms of *anaemia* such as tiredness, breathlessness, angina or heart failure.

Perforation is becoming less frequent, but it has to be remembered as a possible cause of an acute abdomen in a person with a history of 'indigestion'. Perforation may on occasions be the first manifestation of a peptic ulcer.

Malignant change almost never occurs with duodenal ulcers but may be associated with a gastric ulcer. Whether it is a malignant ulcer *de novo* or a malignant change in a benign ulcer is uncertain.

What to do ?

Assessment

The questions to be posed in assessing patients with peptic ulcers are:

(1) Are symptoms due to a peptic ulcer? Is an ulcer present?
(2) What is the activity of the ulcer? How much disability is being caused?
(3) What is the likely course and outcome in the particular individual?

A diagnosis of peptic ulcer is most usually made on positive findings at a barium meal examination and/or endoscopy. **Blood checks** for possible anaemia and for occult blood in faeces may be indicated.

Analysis of gastric contents for level of acidity is not necessary for assessment of uncomplicated duodenal ulcer. It is, however, necessary to check for hypersecretion of acid when a patient has continuing duodenal ulceration following gastric surgery or when Zollinger-Ellison syndrome is suspected (gastric acid hypersecretion, recurrent ulcer and diarrhoea) due to a non-insulin secreting tumour of the Islets of Langerhans.

Ideally, every patient with suspected gastric ulcer should have endoscopy and biopsy to exclude malignancy, and a repeat endoscopy should be carried out after treatment to ensure that healing has occurred. Since it is only early gastric cancer that is curable, it is essential to pick up a malignant ulcer early, and endoscopy should always be carried out if there is any suspicion of malignancy, especially in patients whose symptoms do not subside after treatment.

Differential diagnosis

Similar collections of symptoms may occur in other disorders that have to be differentiated from peptic ulcers.

'Non-ulcer dyspepsia' is a broad generic label for persons presenting with epigastric pains related to meals and relieved by food and alkalis and with an intermittent periodicity, but in whom no ulcers are found on barium meal examinations. They should be followed up and reassessed and re-examined at intervals, if symptoms persist, because in many a duodenal ulcer will be discovered eventually.

Hiatus hernia has become a more frequent and popular diagnosis since barium meals have been conducted in the head-down position.

Gall bladder disease causes intermittent upper abdominal pains. The attacks of biliary colic may be severe and accompanied by vomiting and collapse. They are quite unrelated to meals and are unrelieved by food or alkalis.

Lesions in the large gut and in particular carcinomata of the caecum and ascending and transverse colon may produce vague pains in the abdomen that can be mistaken for peptic ulcers. The pains tend to be central and not epigastric. They are usually colicky and associated with distension and there is some bowel disturbance in most instances.

Anxiety-depression in the non-coping vulnerable individual may lead to various somatic symptoms which may be mistaken for peptic ulcers. The symptoms tend to be vague such as a flatulent-type dyspepsia with a constant ache across the whole of the upper abdomen.

Management

> Aims of treatment:
>
> • relieve symptoms
> • heal the ulcer
> • prevent recurrence
> • prevention of complications.

The most acceptable management of peptic ulcers is that which is successful in relieving symptoms, is simple and least unpleasant to follow, achieves most satisfactory results and is most economic.

Treatment must not be made arduous by over-strict advice on habits, on diet and on medication.

Current medical treatment is effective in achieving the first two aims, of limited value in preventing a recurrence (surgery may be more successful here), and of no value in preventing complications.

(1) *Lifestyle and habits:*

Unless there are some very gross faults in habits, an individual's established lifestyle should not be interfered with without good and proven reasons.

Excessive smoking and drinking of alcohol and lack of exercise are generally accepted as being harmful and on general principles advice should be given to cut or increase respectively.

Smoking reduces the rate of healing of peptic ulcer with treatment, and also leads to more frequent relapses. Smokers should therefore be strongly advised to stop.

Alcohol may damage the gastric mucosa and patients should therefore be advised to moderate their drinking, especially avoiding spirits on an empty stomach.

It is less than reasonable to give advice on occupation, leisure pursuits and hobbies, social and professional activities, unless one is certain that any changes will be beneficial.

(2) *Rest and bed-rest:*

Bed-rest used to be recommended but it carries more risks than benefits. However, during a severe bout a short period of bed-rest may relieve symptoms.

A break away from stressful work for a short period may be helpful in the early stages, but it should not be accepted as regular escape therapy for those with personal problems.

(3) *Diet and drugs:*

The only proven beneficial components of a diet regime are frequent small meals, avoidance of foodstuffs that are thought to produce exacerbations and possibly milk to relieve abdominal pain. Rigid adherence to diet sheets promotes anxiety and excessive self-concern.

Frequent small meals buffer excess gastric acid in duodenal ulcer and should therefore be encouraged. Bedtime snacks should be avoided as this may stimulate nocturnal gastric acid secretion.

Avoid NSAIDs if possible because of their possible reduction of the protective effect of the prostaglandins in the gastric mucus, which might impair ulcer healing.

If NSAIDs are considered necessary, then protection against the development of gastric ulcer can be provided by combination with an H_2 receptor blocker, or more effectively still by misoprostol, a prostaglandin analogue.

(4) *Alkalis and antacids:*

Antacids and alkalis are often effective in controlling the pain in peptic ulcers.

The type of preparation does not appear to matter very much and the simpler it is the better, e.g. magnesium trisilicate or aluminium hydroxide.

They should be taken when the pain is present and in sufficient quantities to control symptoms.

(5) *Antispasmodics:*

It has been assumed that some of the pain of peptic ulcers is caused by muscle spasm and therefore various antispasmodics have been recommended.

Pirenzipine (Gastrozepin), a selective anti-cholinergic drug, may speed ulcer healing, but in general antispasmodic treatment is disappointing.

(6) *Psychotropic drugs:*

Many persons suffering from peptic ulcers are tense and anxious and suffering from effects of recurrent and continuing bouts of pain.

They may also be tense, anxious and depressed for other reasons. It was customary to treat patients with peptic ulcers with sedatives, tranquillizers or anti-depressants. The indications and choice must be left to each individual physician in his assessment of his own patient.

(7) *Carbenoxolone and deglycyrrhizinized liquorice:*

These preparations have been shown to speed the rate of radiographic healing in gastric ulcers and they deserve a trial in patients with gastric ulcers in whom symptoms persist in spite of simple measures with diet and antacids.

Their use is limited by the frequency of side-effects, especially fluid retention with oedema.

(8) *H$_2$-blockers:*

The two original H$_2$-blockers, cimetidine (Tagamet) and ranitidine (Zantac), are effective in healing 80% of ulcers within 4 weeks of starting treatment, and 90% within 8 weeks. The drugs can be given either twice daily or the total dose can be given at night.

Both drugs are equally effective in healing ulcers. Maintenance treatment can be continued at half dose taken every night, for a minimum period of 3 months. Both drugs have been found to be safe after long-term treatment, and the initial anxiety about the possibility of gastric malignancy developing after long-term reduction of gastric acidity has fortunately not been realized. Side-effects may occur:

• drug interactions, e.g. with warfarin, phenytoin
• gynaecomastia – especially with cimetidine
• mental confusion in the elderly
• bone marrow suppression – rare.

There appears to be no significant clinical advantages in using the newer H$_2$-blockers – nizadipine (Axid) and famotidine (Pepsid).

Omeprazole (Losec) is the most potent inhibitor of gastric acid secretion available, and may be used for short periods in patients with peptic ulcer resistant to conventional H$_2$-blockers. Omeprazole is not an H$_2$-blocker but acts by inhibiting an enzyme – hydrogen/potassium ATP-ase – necessary in the secretion of gastric acid.

Other medical treatment:

There are two other drugs which are as effective as H$_2$-blockers in healing ulcers, and may also lead to fewer relapses after treatment.

Bismuth preparation (tripotassium dicitratobismuthate, DeNol). The drug may cause dark stools which could be mistaken for melaena. The mode of action of DeNol is not known, but it may be related to its ability to kill *Helicobacter pylori.*

Sucralfate (a complex of aluminium hydroxide and sulphated sucrose). Mode of action still unclear. Main side-effect is constipation.

(9) *Surgery*:

The choice of surgery as treatment has been left to the last. This is intentional. It is a highly successful therapy in appropriate cases, but it has a mortality rate of 0.1 to 1%, depending on the unit and surgeon.

There are some side-effects and complications in all surgical operations, even with the newer forms of selective vagotomy. Malabsorption leading to anaemia, bone disease and vitamin deficiencies, diarrhoea, dumping and allied symptoms are possible aftermaths, and late complications such as adhesion, intestinal obstruction are also possibilities.

It is the duty of the personal family physician to know what is available surgically for the patient in his own area. He must know what are the latest surgical operations, which of these his local surgical colleagues are using and with what results. He has to balance the severity of symptoms, their persistence and frequency; he has to assess the overall disability produced by the peptic ulcer; he must know his patient and be able to protect him from the surgeon on occasions and to encourage and advise surgery on other occasions.

It is likely that some 10% of patients with *duodenal ulcer* may be resistant to medical therapies. These include those whose onset is in teens or early 20s, with a long history and a family history of ulceration.

With *gastric ulcer* decisions on surgery should be less restrictive and frequent recurrences, non-healing (on endoscopy) and uncertain biopsy reports of possible pre-malignancy all make surgery a possibility.

Complications such as bleeding, perforation and pyloric stenosis may require surgery.

Types of surgical procedures:

- vagotomy plus pyloroplasty for duodenal ulcers
- gastrectomy (Billroth I) for gastric ulcers.

Practical points

- Diagnosis of duodenal or gastric ulcer must be confirmed by barium meal and/or endoscopy.
- Incidence has gone down in the past 20 years but even now annual incidence of 5 new cases per 2000. There may be as many as 100 patients with a past history.
- Duodenal ulcers tend to begin at 20–40 years, gastric ulcers at 50–60
- Natural history is for possible recurrences for 10–15 years, and then for remission.
- Troublesome symptoms/complications: bleeding (10–15%) and perforation (1–2%).
- Occasional symptoms can often be self-controlled by antacids.
- H_2-blockers effective but recurrences are common.
- Surgery may be indicated in 10% of resistant-recurrent cases.

CHAPTER **23**

THE ACUTE ABDOMEN

What is it?

Acute abdominal pain is the principal surgical emergency for the GP, and it is important to make the right decisions, especially in a child where any delay can result in a seriously ill child with peritonitis.

Note that there may also be medical causes for 'the acute abdomen'.

The 'acute abdomen' is a clinical situation that demands urgent action by the physician. It is a collection of conditions which may have in common one or more of the following:

- abdominal pain;
- vomiting;
- shock or collapse;
- serious risks to life.

The acute abdomen demands considerable skill in diagnosis and assessment and in decisions on management, although the actual technical care usually is carried out by a surgeon.

Possible causes

The following is a check-list of possible causes. Most are rare in general practice, but nevertheless should be considered when appropriate.

Their respective rates are shown overleaf.

Surgical causes

- *Inflammatory*:
  acute appendicitis
  acute diverticulitis
  acute cholecystitis
  acute pancreatitis
  acute salpingitis
- *Acute obstruction*:
  intestinal, e.g. strangulated hernia
  biliary ducts – gallstones
  ureters – renal stones
- *Perforated viscus*:
  duodenal/gastric ulcer
  intestine – traumatic
  Fallopian tube – ectopic gestation
- *Intra-abdominal haemorrhage*:
  ruptured ectopic gestation
  traumatic rupture of the spleen
- *Torsion*:
  sigmoid volvulus
  volvulus of the caecum
  twisted ovarian cyst
- *Vascular*:
  dissecting aneurysm
  ruptured abdominal aortic aneurysm

Medical causes

- *Pulmonary* – pleurisy due to:
  pulmonary infection
  pulmonary infarction
  malignant infiltration
- *Cardiac*: myocardial infarction – this is very rare, either in
  hospital or in general practice.
- *Neurological*:
  Bornholm disease
  tabes dorsalis – now rare
  acute lead poisoning, e.g. in battery workers
- Diabetic ketosis
- Haemolytic crisis in sickle cell anaemia

Who gets what and when?

Although 60 persons will consult each year (per 2000) with abdominal pains, only 10 will be possible 'acute abdomens' requiring decisions on possible urgent life-saving actions such as admissions for surgery.

This means that in a professional career of 40 years a GP can expect to deal with 400 cases.

The proportions of the various conditions are shown in Table 23.1 and Figure 23.1.

TABLE 23.1   Acute abdomen – distribution and annual numbers expected in practice of 2000

Condition	%	Annual numbers per 2000
Acute appendicitis	33	3
Colics: renal, biliary	30	3
Intestinal obstruction	10	1
Gynaecological/obstetric	6	1 every 2 years
Peptic ulcers: bleeds/perforation	5	1 every 2 years
Diverticulitis	5	1 every 2 years
Herniae	3	1 every 3 years
Pancreatitis	2	1 every 5 years
Others: medical and surgical	6	1 every 2 years
Total	100%	10

The age and sex distributions differ with the various disorders as shown in Figures 23.2–23.5:

- *Acute appendicitis* (Figure 23.2) is a condition of young adults but, of course, can occur at any age.
- Complications of *herniae* (Figure 23.3) is obstruction and strangulation occurs in male infants and elderly men.
- *Intestinal obstruction* (Figure 23.4) from tumours, adhesions, torsions, etc. increase with age.
- *Colics* (Figure 23.5) are most prevalent (renal and biliary) in the middle-aged.

How do they present?

Whilst minor acute gastro-intestinal infections and disorders occur many times more often than acute abdominal emergencies, unless the possibility of the latter is ever-present in differential diagnosis than serious mistakes will be made.

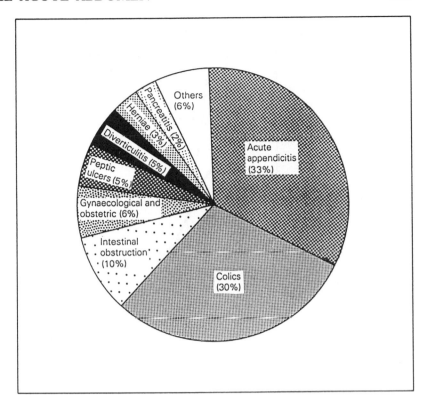

Fig. 23.1—Acute abdomen – distribution

Pointers to the acute abdomen are:

- any abdominal pain that persists for longer than 6 hours
- abdominal tenderness or other abnormal signs
- degrees of general disturbance, i.e. fever, pulse rate, or shock
- special care should be taken at extremes of age when symptoms and signs may be out of keeping with the pathology.

A routine has to be established and followed that must include at the very least an abdominal examination, including hernial orifices, and when indicated a rectal and vaginal examination. Attention must be paid to normal habits such as bowel movements, micturition and menstruation.

Common diseases occur most commonly and acute appendicitis is the most common single cause of the acute abdomen, but there

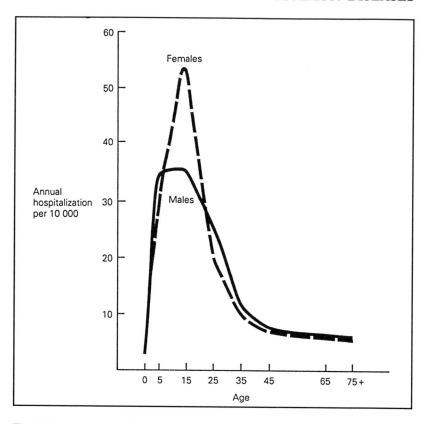

Fig. 23.2—Acute appendicitis – age incidence rates (DHSS, 1978)

are many other possible causes. It is sensible to begin one's clinical approach by considering acute appendicitis as a possible diagnosis and to go on from there.

Clues on examination

- Previous laparotomy scar – consider adhesions with obstruction.
- Hernial orifices for strangulation.
- Distension/peristalsis – consider obstruction.
- Increased bowel sounds – consider obstruction.
- No bowel sounds – consider peritonitis with ileus.
- Rectal examination –
  pelvic tenderness → salpingitis
  pelvic mass
  faecal impaction → obstruction.

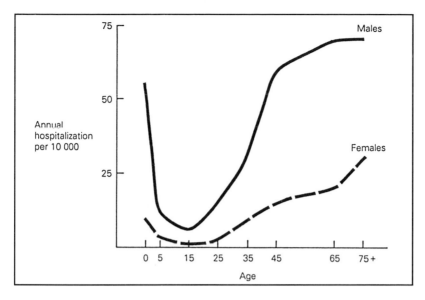

Fig. 23.3—Herniae – age incidence rates (DHSS, 1978)

What happens?

Note that 4000 persons in the UK die from various types of 'acute abdomen' each year during the acute stages.

The course and outcome will depend on the condition and complications.

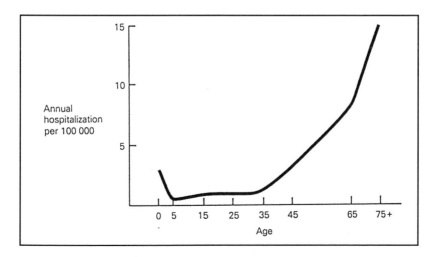

Fig. 23.4—Intestinal obstruction – age incidence rates (DHSS, 1978)

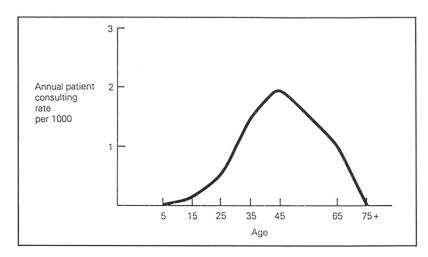

Fig. 23.5—Colics (renal and biliary) – age incidence rates (RCGP/OPCS, 1986)

Thus, whilst early removal of an acutely inflamed *appendix* should be uneventful, delay can lead to a very stormy course with local abscess or general peritonitis and even death in the very young or old.

The outcomes in *intestinal obstruction* depend on the underlying cause, age and condition of the patient.

Perforation or bleeding in *peptic ulcers* carry appreciable mortality rates.

Diverticulitis with perforation occurring in the elderly carries high risks in morbidity and mortality.

What to do?

Assessment

In primary care the first priority is not to make a brilliant definitive pre-operative diagnosis. Rather the physician of first contact must decide on the following:

(1) Has my patient got an 'acute abdomen'?
(2) Should he be hospitalized at once, with a view to surgery?
(3) If not –

- Should further investigations be done, i.e. urine, blood, X-rays?
- Should a second opinion be arranged?
- When should the patient be reassessed?

(4) Whatever is decided, a clear explanation of the reasons for the decision should be given to the patient and the family, as well as possible diagnoses

Diagnostic difficulties in the acute abdomen

- *Infant*:
  history may be difficult to obtain from parents
  examination difficult
  rapid deterioration if undiagnosed.
- *Elderly patients*:
  history may be unclear
  high pain threshold so they do not complain
  unusual presentations, e.g. appendicitis presenting as an acute obstruction.

Investigations which may be helpful in diagnosis include:

- *Urine*:
  may show pyuria in pyelitis
  haematuria in renal stone
  pyuria may also occur in pelvic or retrocaecal appendicitis.
- *Blood count*:
  a raised white cell count supports the diagnosis of appendicitis (it can be normal)
- *Serum amylase*:
  increases + + in acute pancreatitis
  also increases in perforated peptic ulcer and sometimes after a morphine injection.
- *X-ray abdomen*:
  subphrenic gas suggests perforation
  distended fluid-filled loops suggest intestinal obstruction
  radio-opaque renal stones (also mixed or Ca-containing gallstones).
- *Ultrasound*:
  renal stones
  gallstones
- *Chest X-ray*: basal pneumonia with pleurisy.
- *ECG/enzymes*: myocardial infarction.
- *Blood sugar*: diabetic ketosis.

Management

The proper management of a possible acute abdomen is not to take chances. It is much better to admit patients for observation under hospital conditions with access to modern surgical facilities for a short period than to leave the patient unobserved at home.

An accurate specific diagnosis of the acute abdomen is always retrospective and often following laparotomy.

The management of the acute abdomen calls for more skill, experience and application of sound diagnostic methods in primary care than most other situations.

It is not possible to state simply the management procedures to be followed. Each has to develop his, or her, own. The management is largely diagnostic and decision-making.

At first contact with a possible acute abdomen the possibility has to be realized. If a major condition is considered to be likely then, except perhaps with the colics, there is no place for home care. If the diagnosis of an acute abdomen is uncertain then a re-examination of the patient is imperative within the next few hours – there is no place for leaving the patient till the next day.

Practical points

- A GP with 2000 patients will see 60 patients with abdominal pain – 10 of these will be possible 'acute abdomen'.
- Of acute abdomens the most prevalent conditions are acute appendicitis, 3 per year; biliary or renal colics, 3 per year; and intestinal obstruction, 1 per year.
- Acute abdomen is a potentially life-threatening condition.
- There may be considerable difficulties for the GP in diagnosis and management.
- The GP's tasks are not to try and make a precise definitive pathological diagnosis but to decide:
    Is it an 'acute abdomen'?
    Should patient be admitted at once to hospital?
    If not, what further investigations may be appropriate (by GP) and how frequently should the case be reviewed?
- The lesson must be to play safe and take no chances – it is much safer for the patient to be admitted with a negative (no 'acute abdomen') outcome than to sit on a case, delay and risk serious intra-abdominal complications and death.

CHAPTER 24

GALL BLADDER, LIVER AND PANCREAS

What are they?

Diseases of gall bladder, liver and pancreas are not common clinically in primary care – contrary to hospital experience.

Of those that do occur, gallstones and their effects, hepatitis and pancreatic cancer are most prominent.

Who gets them and when?

The annual prevalence rates, from J.F.'s experience, are shown in Table 24.1.

However, autopsy rates reveal that 1 in 5 men and 1 in 3 women have 'silent' gallstones which did not cause any clinical problems.

Annual cholecystectomy rate is 1–2 per GP (with 2000 patients) or 5–10 per group with 10000.

How do they present?

Gallstones

Three types of gallstones are recognized:

- pigment – calcium and bilirubin
- cholesterol
- mixed – cholesterol and bilirubin.

253

TABLE 24.1   Gall bladder, liver and pancreas disorders: annual patient consulting rates

Disorder	Annual consulting rates	
	per 2000	per 10 000
Gall bladder		
Gall stones	2	10
Cholecystitis & possible		
gall bladder dyspepsia	3	15
Liver		
Hepatitis (acute)	less than 1	4
Hepatitis (chronic)		
and cirrhosis	1 in 5 years	1
Pancreas		
Cancer	1 in 5 years	1
Pancreatitis	1 in 5 years	1
Total	6–7	32

Basic causal factors are stasis, infection and alterations in bile content and metabolism.

Increased incidence over the past 50 years is possibly related to diet, overweight, and also related to increased levels of oestrogens in women from medication.

The two main *acute* presentations of gallstones are:

- biliary colic – due to impaction of the stone in the cystic duct
- acute cholecystitis – occurs if the stone remains impacted.

If repeated attacks of acute cholecystitis occur, then a pathological condition of *chronic cholecystitis* may develop. It is very unlikely that the so-called 'gall-bladder dyspepsia', or flatulent dyspepsia, consisting of vague epigastric discomfort, belching, flatulence and intolerance of fatty food, is caused by chronic cholecystitis, since it almost invariably persists following cholecystectomy.

Other associations which may occur as a result of gallstones are:

- *Acute pancreatitis* – this can be a life-threatening acute abdominal emergency; the diagnostic test is the level of serum amylase, which is usually, but not invariably, very high in this condition.
- *Carcinoma of gall bladder* – this is a rare complication but may occur even if the gallstones are silent.

Diagnosis of gallstones

- *Plain X-ray of the abdomen* – radio-opaque mixed stones may be seen in 30% of patients with gallstones.
- *Abdominal ultrasound* – this is the best test for showing gall stones irrespective of their radio-opacity to X-rays.
- *Oral cholecystogram* – identifies 70% of gallstones, not feasible if patient is jaundiced. A poorly functioning gallbladder is not significant in this test because 50% of these are eventually shown to be normal.
- *ERCP* (endoscopic retrograde cholangio-pancreatography) is a valuable new technique, because as well as diagnosing 85% of jaundiced patients due to gallstones, it offers the possibility of gallstone removal at the same time.

Management of gallstones

- *Silent gallstones* – most surgeons recommend elective prophylactic cholecystectomy because of the possibility of complications, including carcinoma of the gall bladder in the future, but note the high autopsy rates of silent gallstones that did not cause problems.
  Operation has a 0.5% mortality (2% in the elderly).
- *Biliary colic* – elective cholecystectomy.
- *Acute cholecystitis* – conservative initially; subsequent elective cholecystectomy.

Other methods of treating gallstones

- Medical dissolution of stones with oral bile salts (cheno-deoxycholic acid) – may take up to 2 years to dissolve completely. Unfortunately, the stones recur in most patients within a few years. It is unsuitable for calcified or pigment stones. This treatment is falling out of favour.
- Shockwave lithotripsy – stones are shattered and excreted via the cystic duct.
- Mechanical crushing of gallstones through a catheter introduced at radiology (ERCP) or on laparoscopy.

Viral hepatitis

Five main viruses are now recognized to cause viral hepatitis

(1) *Hepatitis A* –

- transmitted via oral/faecal route [incubation rate 30 days];
- primarily affects adults – clinical disease;

- is rare in infants and young children, except in developing countries.

(2) *Hepatitis B*
  - spread by percutaneous, permucosal and intravenous routes;
  - mean incubation period 75 days;
  - risk factors:
    male homosexuality
    intravenous drugs
    low socio-economic status
    sexual promiscuity
    mental institutions
    health professions.

(3) *Hepatitis C* (nonA-nonB) – responsible for post-transfusion hepatitis – occurs in 2–10% of patients having multiple transfusions.
  - risk factors:
    haemodialysis patients
    transplant – kidney
                 bone marrow
                 liver
                 i.v. drugs
                 male homosexuals
                 ? perinatal transmission

(4) *Hepatitis D*
  - only affects patients already infected with hepatitis B;
  - transmitted by parenteral route.

(5) *Hepatitis E* – predominantly in developing countries.

Clinical features of acute viral hepatitis

Clinical features are similar in all types of acute viral hepatitis – only the epidemiological factor and the different incubation periods serve to distinguish between them.

- *Symptoms*
  Usually insidious onset with malaise, anorexia and discomfort in the right hypochondrium.
  Additional symptoms in hepatitis B include –
  fever
  arthralgia
  urticaria.
- Onset of jaundice after a few days, though the jaundice may occur *de novo* without any preceding symptoms – when the jaundice appears the other symptoms may improve.

The jaundice may last from a few days to several months –   the average is 2–3 weeks.
With the onset of jaundice –
itching
pale stools
weight loss
children with type B hepatitis may develop a papular rash.

- *Physical signs*
low-grade fever
jaundice
mild tender liver enlargement
mild splenomegaly (5–10%)
enlarged glands
- *Liver function tests*
serum aminotransferases – increased × 10 – 50; if the levels remain high for over 6 months then the likelihood of progressive liver disease is high
bilirubin increased
alkaline phosphatase only mildly increased
serum albumin usually normal
prothrombin increased
blood count normal
serological diagnosis should be made if possible.

Management

- Most patients can be treated at home.
- Admission is necessary if –
social reasons
diagnosis in doubt
prothrombin time very prolonged.
If admitted barrier nursing is desirable.
- Stop all unnecessary drugs, e.g. NSAIDs, contraceptives.
- No specific treatment is usually necessary – bed rest is necessary only if the patient is jaundiced or is otherwise symptomatic.
- No alcohol for at least 6–12 months.
- Interferon may be tried in severe cases.
- Liver biopsy is unnecessary unless the diagnosis is uncertain.

Note: availability of hepatitis B immunization for at-risk groups and for infants and children in high prevalence countries.

Outcome of viral hepatitis

- Hepatitis A doesn't usually progress to chronic hepatitis.

- Hepatitis B
  may lead to liver failure with fulminant hepatitis
  may be asymptomatic in many patients
  may progress to chronic hepatitis
  liver carcinoma can develop in patients with chronic hepatitis.
- Hepatitis C
  may progress to fulminant hepatitis
  50% develop chronic liver disease – may take up to 10 years
  liver carcinoma is possible.
- Hepatitis D occurs with hepatitis B so this determines the prognosis.
- Hepatitis E
  high mortality – 20%
  associated with a high incidence of disseminated intravascular coagulation, especially if it affects pregnant women.

Pancreatitis and cancer of pancreas

Pancreatitis acute and chronic is rare in practice – one new case every 5 years.

Acute pancreatitis is an acute abdominal emergency with pain and collapse, and associated with gallstones and high alcohol intake.

Chronic pancreatitis is less dramatic with bouts of upper abdominal pain and effects of damage to the gland leading to dyspepsia, malabsorption and diabetes.

Cancer of pancreas also is uncommon and presents gradually with weight loss, vague dyspepsia, jaundice and backache. Beware of jaundice persisting and increasing for over 2 weeks in any patient.

What happens?

Gallstones

Many gallstones are silent and do not seem to cause clinical problems.

Once they do so then they are likely to continue with recurrent biliary colic and possible jaundice.

Hepatitis

As noted, hepatitis A usually resolves naturally without much risk of chronic hepatitis. The chances of chronic hepatitis and even hepatic cancer are greater in hepatitis B and C.

Pancreatitis

- Acute pancreatitis has an appreciable mortality rate.
- Chronic pancreatitis is a persisting disorder.

Pancreatic cancer has a low (less than 5%) 5-year survival rate.

What to do?

The particular roles of the primary physician in this group of conditions are:

- As early diagnosis as possible based on clinical suspicions supported by investigations.
- With *gall bladder diseases* a decision in each case as to whether to refer the patient for elective surgical procedures.
- Consideration of active immunization against hepatitis B for at-risk occupational groups such as doctors, nurses, dentists, paramedics, police and fire service workers, or for children in high prevalence areas.

Practical points

- Although as many as 1 in 4 adults have gallstones few will develop significant clinical problems.
- Cholecystectomy cures biliary colic attacks but may not relieve 'gall bladder dyspepsia'.
- The various types of hepatitis viruses are increasing in number but hepatitis is uncommon in practice – most prevalent is hepatitis A which resolves without serious after-effects; hepatitis B potentially is more serious and active immunization should be considered for at-risk groups.
- Painless jaundice persisting for more than 2 weeks may be due to cancer of pancreas.

CHAPTER 25

CANCERS OF THE GASTRO-INTESTINAL TRACT

What are they?

Cancers of the gastro-intestinal (GI) tract are the most prevalent site of neoplasia – they account for one-quarter of all cancers. The clinical features depend on the site affected and the mechanical effects produced. Unfortunately prognosis still is poor but early and even presymptomatic diagnosis and treatment improve outlook for surgical excision which is the only potentially effective treatment at present.

Who gets what, where and when?

Table 25.1 shows the annual incidence of new cases of gastro-intestinal cancers in practices of 2000 and 10 000 population bases.

The incidence increases with age from 40 onwards and men are more likely to be affected.

TABLE 25.1   Cancers of gastro-intestinal tract: annual new cases

Site	New cases	
	per 2000	per 10 000
Oesophagus	1 in 8 years	1 in 2 years
Stomach	1 in 3 years	1–2 per year
Colon	1 in 2 yreas	2–3 per year
Rectum	1 in 3 years	1–2 per year
Pancreas	1 in 5 years	1 per year
Liver and gall bladder	1 in 8 years	1 in 2 years
Total	3 every 2 years	7–8 per year

How do they present?

The earliest features are those of relatively minor functional disturbance.

Thus with *oesophageal cancer*, food may 'stick' in the chest, at first only with meat. In *stomach cancer* the earliest symptoms are 'indigestion' with vague epigastric discomfort, flatulence with an unpleasant taste, anorexia, loss of weight and general malaise.

Cancer of the caecum is often 'silent' with anaemia as the presenting sign, a mass may be felt in the right iliac fossa and there may be a vague lower abdominal discomfort with loose stools.

Cancer of the colon presents with altered bowel habits, constipation and/or diarrhoea and bouts of colicky abdominal pains. A mass may be palpable – but this is usually a late sign.

Cancer of the rectum presents with passage of blood per rectum, loose stools mixed with blood and mucus. Urgency of defaecation or a feeling of incomplete passage of stools may be noted. A mass or ulcer may be felt on rectal examination.

Cancer of the pancreas, liver or gall bladder most often presents with obstructive jaundice, loss of weight and backache.

Clinical features

Carcinoma of stomach

Cancer of stomach is the third commonest carcinoma in the UK (behind lung and colon). It is almost invariably an adenocarcinoma.

Possible causal factors

- Blood group A.
- High salt intake.

- Living in areas with high nitrate content in the soil – bacterial breakdown leads to the formation of nitrosamines which are carcinogenic.
- Certain occupations, e.g. rubber processing.
- Chronic gastritis may predispose, e.g. chronic atrophic gastritis in pernicious anaemia.
- Subtotal gastric resection – predisposes to chronic gastritis.

Symptoms

- Early cases often asymptomatic.
- Ulcer pain may occur with a less defined relationship to meals.
- Symptoms of iron-deficiency anaemia.
- General – anorexia, weight loss.

Signs

- Abdominal mass.
- Enlarged liver due to metastases.
- Enlarged supraclavicular glands (Trousseau's sign).
- Ascites.

Investigations

- Barium meal.
- Endoscopy – a more useful test because of the possibility of biopsy.
- CT scanning – especially useful in detecting hepatic and lymph node metastases.
- Endoscopic ultrasound – new technique for outlining layers of gastric wall – can show the depth of invasion of the tumour.

Management

Surgery offers the only hope of cure if the cancer is diagnosed early – the 5-year survival can be as high as 90% if the condition is detected early enough. In more advanced cancer the 5-year survival is only 10% and this has not changed much in the last 25 years.

Surgery can also offer palliative bypass operation if obstruction occurs.

Chemotherapy can prolong life by a few months, but only 40% of patients respond.

Carcinoma of the colon

The commonest type of gastro-intestinal malignancy in the developed world. It is seldom seen in developing countries.

Possible causal factors

- Dietary factors may be relevant – high fat, low fibre.
- Colonic polyps – most colon cancer develops from benign adenomatous polyps. Polyps are found in 35% of operated cases.
- There may be a genetic factor linked to chromosome 5.

Symptoms

- Rectal bleeding in patients over 40 years of age is the commonest manifestation and requires urgent investigation.
- Colicky left-sided abdominal pain.
- Alteration in bowel habits – diarrhoea, constipation or both.
- Tenesmus.
- Symptoms due to iron-deficiency anaemia.

Signs

- Abdominal mass – tumour mass or enlarged liver.
- Rectal mass.
- Evidence of obstruction with distension, increased peristalsis and increased bowel sounds.

Investigations

- Faecal occult blood tests – 50% sensitivity in picking up carcinoma of GI tract.
- Sigmoidoscopy with biopsy prior to barium studies.
- Barium enema – 10% of cancers and 20% of polyps may be missed.
- Colonoscopy – best test for cancer of colon.

Management

- *Polyps* – remove through a colonoscope.
- *Carcinoma* – surgery is the best treatment. In District General Hospitals only 50% are found to be suitable for radical surgery and among these the 5-year survival is only 30%.
- Cytotoxic treatment has been found of doubtful benefit, but may be useful for treatment of metastases: a solitary metastasis in the liver can be removed surgically.
- *Follow-up* is essential – every 6 months for at least 5 years and should include:
  clinical assessment
  liver scans for mestastases
  regular estimation of carcinoembryonic antigen – a chemical marker for the presence of colonic carcinoma.

What happens?

The general outlook is not good but varies with site and stage of the disease.

5-year survival rates for all grades of the various sites are:

Five-year survival rates	
Oesophagus	8%
Stomach	10%
Colon	35%
Rectum	36%
Pancreas, liver and gall bladder	less than 5%

What to do?

The physician of first contact has the difficult task of picking out the potentially serious gastro-intestinal conditions, such as the cancers, from the mass of minor functional disorders.

It is no easy task. There are no definitive reliable features. Any symptoms that do not clear within a few weeks should be taken as potentially serious and investigated radiologically and endos-copically in collaboration with specialists.

The general management of these patients is difficult because their outlook is so poor and the patient and the family will need much care and support over some years.

The primary physician has to think of the likely diagnosis and put into train the sequence of events from confirmation of diagnosis to definitive treatment, after care and, sadly, often terminal care.

Hope for better prognosis lies in screening in order to pick out early cases.

Screening for cancer of the GI tract

Screening for cancer of the gastro-intestinal tract is worth considering in those patients who are at particular risk.

Oesophagus

- 5000 patients die of oesophageal cancer annually in the UK.
- Predisposing factors
  achalasia of the cardia
  coeliac disease
  Plummer-Vincent syndrome.

- Pre-malignant conditions
  Barrett's oesophagus
  chronic oesophagitis.
- Methods
  oesophagoscopy and biopsy – picks up 90% of the cases –   best
   screening method
  barium swallow – misses small lesions.

Stomach

All patients with new onset of indigestion particularly if an atypical pattern and persistent should be considered for screening for gastric cancer.

- *Predisposing factors*
  pernicious anaemia
  previous gastric resection.
- *Pre-malignant conditions*
  chronic gastritis
  chronic gastric ulcer.
- *Methods*
  gastroscopy and biopsy best
  barium meal
  chemical 'markers' in the blood:
      foetal sulphoglycoprotein
      lactic dehydrogenase (LDH)
      carcino-embryonic antigen;
  cytology in gastric washings.

Colorectal carcinoma

- *Predisposing factors*
  familial polyposis of the colon
  previous colorectral cancer
  colorectal cancer in first degree family relatives.
- *Pre-malignant conditions*
  colorectal adenoma
  long-standing ulcerative colitis (over 10 years).
- *Methods*
  endoscopy and biopsy best
  barium enema
  faecal occult blood tests.

Practical points

- A group practice of 10 000 can expect 7–8 new cases of GI tract cancer each year.
- Stomach, colon and rectum are most likely sites.
- In general, 5-year overall survival rate of GI cancers is 30% but better in stomach and colorectal cases that are diagnosed early.

SECTION V

RHEUMATIC DISEASES

CHAPTER 26

MUSCULO-SKELETAL AND CONNECTIVE TISSUE DISORDERS – THE CLINICAL SPECTRUM

To use a more homely title, 'rheumatism' is a frequent cause of disability in the community (over one-third of all severely disabled). Although it is not often a life-threatening disorder it accounts for much work in general practice.

The term 'rheumatism' is helpful and justifiable because the conditions that are included cover a wide range of clinical syndromes most of which are of unknown or uncertain cause. A common sense pragmatic approach to classification and management is necessary.

As will be seen, the clinical spectrum includes systematic conditions such as rheumatoid arthritis, gout and rarities not mentioned by name such as various anthropathies and local manifestations of joint and soft tissue pathologies.

Classification based on accurate knowledge of pathology and definitive causation is not possible because of lack of understanding; therefore rather vague and imprecise labels have to be acceptable.

Patients consulting

In a year 13% of the practice population consult for these conditions (Table 26.1). This represents almost 1 in 5 of all those who actually consult during a year. The rate is higher for females (15%) than males (12%). One-third are graded as 'severe' and one-half as 'trivial' (Third National Morbidity Survey).

Taken as a group, prevalence increases with age (Figure 26.1).

TABLE 26.1 Musculo-skeletal and connective tissue disorders – consultation rates increase with age

	Age – years							
	0–4	5–14	15–24	25–44	45–64	65–74	75+	All
Annual patients consulting per 1000	17	41	82	135	200	222	240	133

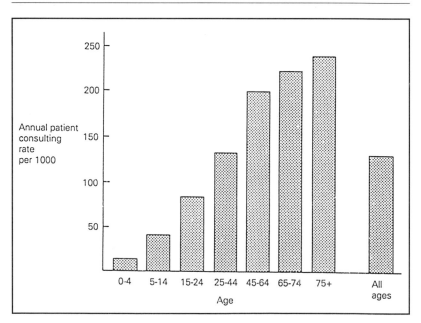

Fig. 26.1—Prevalence of musculo-skeletal and connective tissue disorders increases with age

Table 26.2 shows the numbers of patients who consult in a year in a group practice of 2000 and in a group practice of 10 000, by diagnosis. 'Arthritis' and 'back disorders' are the largest groups but the collection of connective tissue conditions is not far behind.

TABLE 26.2 Annual consultation rates for musculo-skeletal and connective tissue disorders

	Patients consulting	
Disorder	per 2000	per 10 000
Arthritis		
Rheumatoid	12	60
Osteoarthritis	48	240
Vague 'arthritis'	50	250
Gout	6	30
	116	580
Connective tissue		
Shoulder syndromes	14	70
Tendinitis, bursitis, ganglion, etc.	24	120
Other non-articular (muscle, ligament, etc.)	26	130
	64	320
Back disorders		
Back pain	58	290
Osteoarthritis of spine	8	40
Cervical spinal	24	120
Lumber disc, sciatica	20	100
Other back conditions	10	50
	120	600
Other pains in limbs	40	200

Source: Third National Morbidity Survey

Taking the 'back' section in a different dimension, 51% presented as 'acute backs', 34% were 'chronic backs', and 15% 'intermediate'.

Consultations

8.5% of all GP consultations are for 'rheumatic' disorders.

Sickness absence

These conditions account for 12% of all certified sickness absence from work.

Disability

It is difficult to estimate the extent of disability from rheumatic disorders in the community because of different criteria used to define 'disability'.

What is certain is that many, or most, of those 'disabled' do not necessarily consult their GPs frequently and regularly, but appear to accept their disabilities.

- 10% of the population is said to have some disability from osteoarthritis. This means 200 persons in a practice of 2000. However, taking 'osteoarthritis' and 'vague arthritis' from Table 26.2 (98 consultations) these represent less than one-half of those disabled.
- 3% of the population is said to have some disability from 'rheumatoid arthritis'. This means 60 persons in a practice of 2000 but only 12 consult annually (Table 26.2).

In population surveys rheumatic disorders are responsible for one-third of all those severely disabled.

Hospital admissions

Although only 3% of all admissions to hospital are for these disorders, this means 8 patients per practice of 2000 and 40 per group with 10 000 patients. About one-half will be for surgical procedures.

Causes of death

Around 6000 deaths are listed as due to rheumatic diseases. This represents just under 1% (0.94) of all deaths.

CHAPTER **27**

LOW BACKACHE

What is it?

Backache is a universal experience and the consequence of our human two-legged stance and locomotion.

Generally benign in terms of risks to life, yet it is disabling, incapacitating and the cause of much suffering and loss of work time.

Although easy to define symptomatically, its exact causes and pathology are uncertain and unclear. There is poor correlation between symptoms and signs and pathology.

The back is a complex structure of many tissues, each being capable of causing backache alone or in combination.

Although it is possible to differentiate between acute and chronic backache, the two may merge or there may be acute episodes in a chronic sufferer.

The *causes* are many and may be divided conveniently into broad groups and into common and uncommon (Table 27.1.).

Who gets it when?

In general *acute backache* tends to be a condition of active adults. *Chronic backache* tends to occur in inactive adults and late middle age.

273

TABLE 27.1 Backache: causes and frequency

Common	Uncommon
Mechanical	
• Strains, injuries (to muscle, joint, disc)	• Spondylolisthesis
• Osteoarthrosis	• Juvenile osteochondritis
• Spontaneous collapse of vertebra (metabolic or neoplastic)	
Inflammatory	
• Rheumatoid disease	• Polymyalgia
	• Ankylosing spondylitis
	• Osteomyelitis
	• Tuberculosis
Neoplasia	
• Secondary deposits	• Myeloma
	• Spinal tumours
Metabolic	
• Osteoporosis	• Osteomalacia
• Steroid – complications	• Paget's disease
	• Parathyroid disorders
Referred	• Peptic ulcers
	• Gall bladder disease
	• Pancreatic disease
	• Aortic aneurysm
Pelvic disorders (gynaecological)	
• Vaginal prolapse	
• Inflammatory disease	
Uncertain	
• Associated with psychiatric disorders?	
• 'Compensationitis'?	
• Postural?	
• Occupational?	

Backache is a frequent reason for consultation. A GP with 2000 patients can expect to be consulted in a year by patients with

- acute backache 65
- chronic backache 52
- 'back invalids' 3

The *age prevalence* differs in the various groups:
- In children juvenile osteochondritis is rare.
- *Age 15–30*
  - strains and injuries

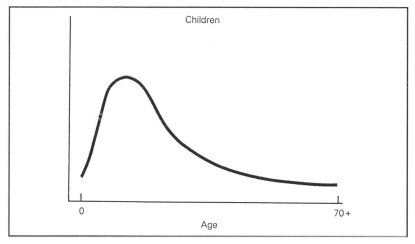

Fig. 27.1—Childhood back problems – age prevalence

- prolapsed intervertebral disc (PID)
- ankylosing spondylitis
- spondylolisthesis
- Age 30–50
  - PID   strains   injuries
  - 'chronic backache'
  - psychiatric?
  - secondary deposits
  - primary spinal tumours

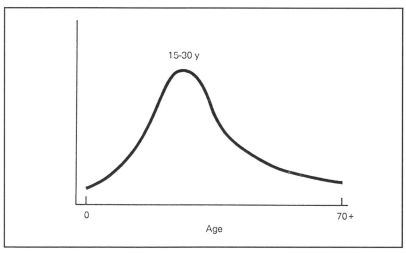

Fig. 27.2—Backache in the 15–30 age group

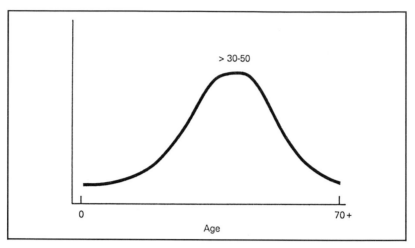

Fig. 27.3—Backache in the 30–50 age group

- *Age over 50*
    - strains
    - chronic backache
    - osteoarthrosis
    - secondary deposits
    - osteoporosis
    - myeloma
    - Paget's disease
    - aneurysms

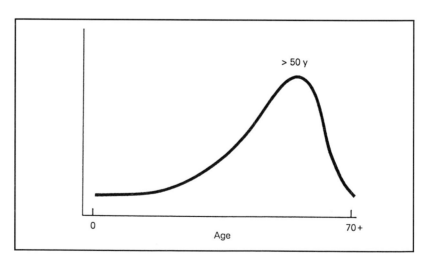

Fig. 27.4—Backache in the over–50s

How do they present?

Most backache is referred to the lower lumbar and lumbo-sacral region.

The *onset* may be acute, subacute or chronic.

Acute

Sudden and often related to a minor twist or lifting. Degrees of disability range from an annoying ache aggravated by movement to severe incapacity with victim being unable to get out of bed. There may be radiation down one leg (sciatica). Rarely with a severe PID there may be interference with micturition and defecation (Figure 27.5).

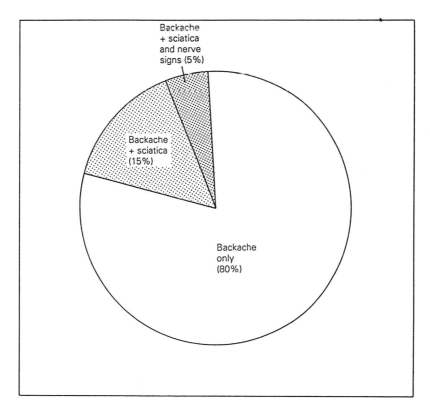

Fig. 27.5—Acute backache

Chronic

> Persistent ache that may be constant or intermittent. Often related to certain positions such as sitting, driving, work.

What happens?

Acute

> Three out of four will recover within 4 weeks whatever the treatment.
>> *Recurrences* are common.

Chronic

> May persist for years but tends to become less after the age of 60 in the non-specific types, presumably because of natural reduction in mobility of back and activity of person.
> *Note* that it is likely that:

> - Only one in 10 of back sufferers consult GP.
> - One in 20 will be referred by the GP to a specialist (hospital).
> - Surgery for only one patient in 5 years per GP.

What to do?

General points to remember

- Backache is very common.
- Most acute attacks will settle on their own within 4 weeks.
- Chronic backache is difficult to manage but this too tends to improve as persons become older – unless caused by some rare and serious underlying disease.
- There are very many treatments available and recommended – none are universally effective for all types or even for one type.

Assessment

> Although most cases are benign and amenable to relief, the challenges to the GP must be:

> - Beware of possible serious causes such as malignant deposits.
> - Consider ankylosing spondylitis in a young man with persistent low backache.

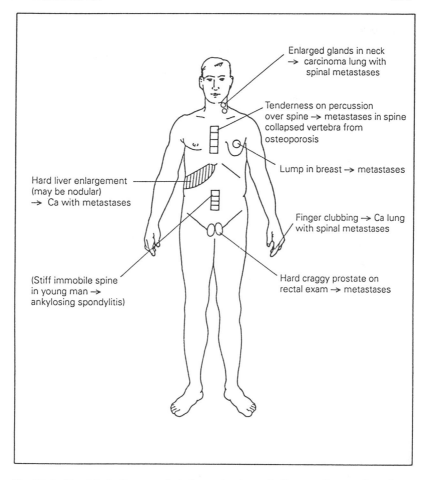

Enlarged glands in neck
→ carcinoma lung with
spinal metastases

Tenderness on percussion
over spine → metastases in spine
collapsed vertebra from
osteoporosis

Lump in breast → metastases

Hard liver enlargement
(may be nodular)
→ Ca with metastases

Finger clubbing → Ca lung
with spinal metastases

(Stiff immobile spine
in young man →
ankylosing spondylitis)

Hard craggy prostate on
rectal exam → metastases

Fig. 27.6—Possible findings on clinical examination to indicate malignancy in patients with low backache

- Acute backache in elderly persons is rarely due to strains or PID – more likely to be associated with underlying pathology such as collapse of vertebra due to osteoporosis or malignancy (consider secondary deposits from lung, breast, prostate cancers).
- Do not label chronic back sufferers as malingerers, psychiatric cases or something similar just because you (and other therapists) cannot help them !

Examination

In addition to the back, check legs, (straight leg raise and reflexes); examine breasts in women and prostate in men; consider possible lung cancer in male smokers or ex-smokers.

Investigations

Routine investigations are not indicated.

Lumbosacral X-ray

This will reveal structural changes such as collapse of vertebra, spondylitis, spondylolisthesis and osteoporosis – which are uncommon causes.

Reduction of disc spaces and osteophytes are 'normal abnormalities' and occur as often in persons without symptoms as in those with backache.

Therefore, be selective in ordering an X-ray. However, it may be necessary to convince a patient that nothing important or treatable has been missed.

Blood ESR

Blood ESR will be raised with myelomata, cancer and inflammatory disorders such as polymyalgia.

Management

It is useful to write out a personal, or a practice protocol:

- *Mild acute attacks* may be treated with advice, reassurance and analgesics.
- *Disabling acute attacks* should be advised bed rest until pain improves.
- *Persisting backache* – where the patient becomes despondent and loses faith, then referral to a physiotherapist may help to relieve tension.
- *Chronic backache* that does not respond to analgesics, NSAIDs and physical forms of therapy may require referral to a specialist more for reassurance than for active therapy.
- *Surgery* can be dramatically successful for a definite PID or spinal stenosis but not so for non-specific chronic backache.

Specific management – comments

Rest in bed is sensible when the victim cannot get out of bed but it is not so sensible for less severe types since it tends to cause muscle weakness and other effects of imposed bed rest such as venous thrombosis and constipation.

Analgesics and NSAIDs should be used in adequate dosage to relieve acute episodes but with more care and discrimination in chronic backache.

Specific disorders such as myeloma, spondylitis, malignancies require specialist care.

Local injections into tender back areas with steroids and local anaesthetics are used and are said to be helpful in some cases, but not in all.

Manipulations have their enthusiastic performers and patients. It is difficult to select appropriate cases.

Spinal supports may be helpful and should not be denied the chronic sufferers.

Surgery as noted should be reserved for the proven PID. Selection of other chronic cases for bone grafting and other measures must be decisions for the super-specialists.

General advice, explanation and support for the individual patient are important and appreciated with attention to hobbies, occupation, weight and exercises.

Practical points

- Backache is a universal complaint. It is of three varieties – acute, recurrent and chronic.
- It is a symptom of many possible causes but the common types are of uncertain causation.
- Most acute attacks are benign, self-limiting and recover naturally within 4 weeks.
- A GP with 2000 patients may expect to see around 120 with backache each year – more than one-half of these will be acute cases. There will be about 3 patients who are 'back invalids' and who are severely disabled long term.
- Although uncommon, a number of serious diseases can cause backache, as neoplasms, usually secondary deposits, or myeloma, osteoporosis with vertebral collapse, spondylitis and polymyalgia.
- Chronic backache with no serious underlying disease tends to improve after 60.
- Management should be commonsensical. First, be aware constantly that there may be serious (rare) causes. Second, beware of labelling persons with backache malingerers or neurotic, although these may be factors.
- Symptomatic treatment with rest when necessary and analgesics is adequate in most acute cases.
- The efficacy of the many other treatments is uncertain but all have their enthusiastic proponents.
- Surgery is indicated only for specific conditions such as proven PID, spinal stenosis or localized tumours.
- The physician's understanding and support are important in chronic cases.

CHAPTER **28**

OSTEOARTHROSIS

What is it?

As we age so do our bodily organs and structures. It is not surprising therefore that intricate joints wear out. Osteoarthritis (or osteoarthrosis) is a 'normal abnormality' involving thinning of cartilage, inflammation of synovia and osteophyte formation.

Whilst radiological evidence of osteoarthrosis in the body is widespread, affecting some joints in almost everyone aged 65 and over, these changes do not necessarily cause symptoms and even when they do, not every person feels the need to consult a GP.

The most likely joints shown to be affected on routine radiological examination of persons over 65 are:

• cervical spine in	22%
• shoulders in	35%
• hands in	66%
• hips in	38%
• knees in	46%
• feet in	49%

Most problems occur when weight-bearing joints such as hips and knees are involved.

283

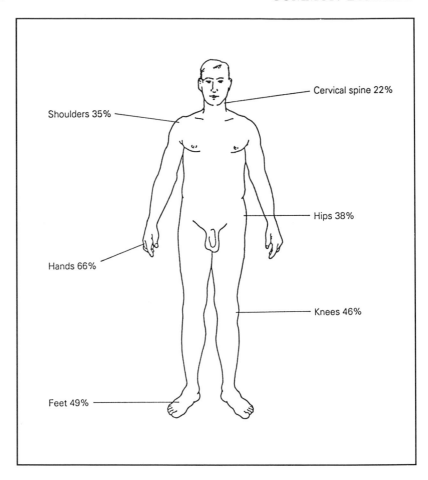

Fig. 28.1—Frequency of joint involvement in osteoarthrosis

Osteoarthrosis is divided into two main types – primary and secondary.

The *primary type* is due to primary degenerative changes in the articular cartilage which occurs as a result of ageing, and is unrelated to any systemic or local disease, although there is some evidence of a hereditary factor.

The *secondary type* of osteoarthrosis is indistinguishable pathologically from the primary type, but results from a variety of underlying causes, such as:

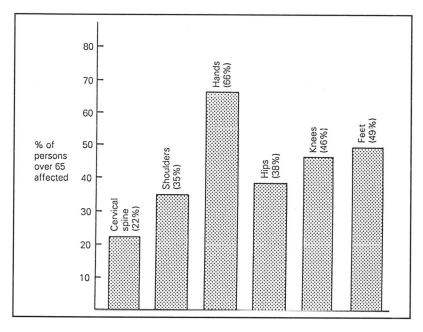

Fig. 28.2—Osteoarthrosis in the over–65s

- trauma, e.g. previous joint fracture
- congenital disorders, e.g. Perthes' disease
- primary joint disease, e.g. rheumatoid arthritis
- endocrine disease, e.g. diabetes, acromegaly
- mechanical reasons, e.g. gross obesity
- others, e.g. repeated haemarthrosis in haemophilia.

Who gets it and when?

As noted the condition is associated with ageing (Figure 28.3). Also noted is the fact that most persons with osteoarthrosis do not consult their GP during a year.

Table 28.1 shows that in a year in a practice of 2000, 48 patients will consult for osteoarthrosis and another 50 for 'arthritis'. Most of these will be over 65. In a practice of 2000, 300 (15%) are over 65. Thus the annual consulting rate in this group for 'arthritis' will be 16% for osteoarthrosis and 17% for 'arthritis', suggesting that 1 in 3 of elderly do consult.

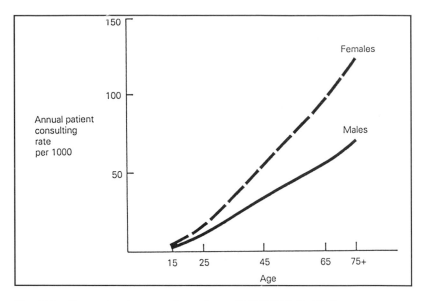

Fig. 28.3—Osteoarthrosis – annual prevalence (RCGP/OPCS, 1986)

TABLE 28.1   Osteoarthrosis: annual consulting rates per 2000 and 10 000 and rates for over 65s

Disorder	Annual persons consulting	
	per 2000	per 10 000
Osteoarthrosis	48	240
Arthritis	50	250
	Rates (%) in over 65s	
	Numbers	%
Osteoarthrosis	48/300	16%
Arthritis	50/300	17%
Total		33%

How do they present?

Symptoms

The *symptoms* can be divided into early and late:

● Early:
pain on movement of the joints, particularly after use
morning stiffness of short duration

night pain
responsive to anti-inflammatory drugs.
- Late:
rest pain
thickening of joints with effusion
joint instability
lack of responsiveness to anti-inflamatory drugs.

Signs

- Few signs early in the disease.
- Later:
crepitus
swelling of the joints – the swelling may be bony or due to effusion
limitation of active and passive movement
joint deformities in hands, knees and feet.

Heberden's nodes

- Bony swellings at the distal interphalangeal joints in the fingers. In the acute stage, the nodes may be acutely inflamed, but subsequently settle down to painless bony swellings often with joint deformity.
- They are more common in women at the menopause or in late middle age.
- Apart from being female, heredity and microtrauma to the distal interphalangeal joints are thought to be aetiological factors.
- Less commonly, similar bony swellings may occur at the proximal interphalangeal joints (Bouchard's nodes).

The other joints which are frequently affected by osteoarthrosis are:

- First carpo-metacarpal joint of the hands.
- *Knees* – this is the most common cause of disability from osteoarthrosis, and is frequently associated with synovial thickening, crepitus and effusion (50% of the patients).
- *Hips* – groin pain on weight-bearing referred to the front of the thigh is a dominant symptom.
- *Spine* – osteoarthrosis is common in the cervical spine and the lumbo-sacral spine. Pain on movement and restriction of joint mobility are common symptoms. In the cervical spine, referral of the pain to the shoulders, arms, fingers and to the interscapular area are frequent: in the lumbo-sacral area, the pain is often referred down the lower limbs in the pattern of sciatica.

Another important though relatively infrequent complication of lumbar osteoarthritis is compression of the spinal canal and cauda equina with the development of the *spinal stenosis syndrome*. This condition may be easily confused with intermittent claudication.

Diagnostic tests for osteoarthrosis

The most useful test is the *X-ray*. This may show:

- narrowing of the joint space
- osteophytes at the margins of the joints
- sclerosis of the underlying bone
- cyst formation can occur
- if the osteoarthrosis is associated with the deposition of pyrophosphate crystals in the joint, linear calcification may be seen.

However, many asymptomatic people over 65 have abnormal X-rays! If there is any suggestion of compression due to lesions of the spine, then a CT scan or a NMR (nuclear magnetic resonance) scan should be carried out.

Blood tests are of no value since there are no abnormalities in ESR, white count or blood biochemistry.

Examination of the *synovial fluid* from an affected joint may be helpful in distinguishing other joint conditions, such as rheumatoid arthritis or pyarthrosis. It is also necessary to confirm a pyrophosphate arthropathy (5% of cases of osteoarthrosis).

What happens?

Osteoarthrosis is not necessarily progressive and disabling. Even when the condition begins to cause symptoms such symptoms may be intermittent with periods of freedom.

Knees and hips are likely to cause most problems with pain and interference with normal functions and it is with these joints that radical surgical procedures must be considered. Hip and knee replacements are now standard procedures when symptoms are severe enough. The decision to operate must be a joint agreement between surgeon and patient.

The *annual rate* for hip *replacement* in the UK is 1–2 per 2000 and that for *knee replacement* (at present) is 0.25–0.5 per 2000.

Since the prevalence of osteoarthritis of the hip in a practice population of 2000 will be 100 (1/3 of 300 persons age 65+) the chances of one of these 100 having a hip replacement over 20 years must be less than 1 in 5.

For knee replacements the chance is only 1 in 15.

What to do?

Management

The management of osteoarthrosis can be divided into the following:

- *General measures* such as weight reduction. When weight bearing joints are affected and avoidance of trauma is necessary, this may mean a change of occupation or giving up traumatic activities.
- *Pain relief* through use of analgesics and trials of anti-inflammatory drugs.
- *Physiotherapy* has a place in relieving acutely reactive joints and in helping to maintain function through muscle exercises.
- *Physical aids* such as splints, walking aids, etc. aid in rehabilitation after surgery.
- *Surgery* now has much to offer in *replacing severely affected joints* such as hips and knees with artificial prostheses. Some progress is being made also in replacement of shoulders and elbows. Selection of patients for joint replacement operations is an individual matter. The chief criteria must be extent of pain and functional disability produced by the damaged joints and the general physical and mental state of the patient and his ability to undertake the procedure and benefit from it. Successful replacement of osteoarthritic joints is one of the most dramatically rewarding of all surgical operations. The patient is relieved of pain and function is restored. Note that the annual rate of joint replacement in the UK is less than 1 per 2500.

There are other *surgical procedures* that may help osteoarthritic joints in selected cases. Arthrodesis – permanent stiffening of joints – may relieve pain but interfere with function. Arthroplasty – artificial joint improvement – may relieve pain and restore function but the results are not as good as joint replacement.

Practical points

- Osteoarthrosis is a wearing out of joints. The most frequently affected joints are in the hands, feet, knees, hips, shoulders and neck. It is a condition of ageing and in the over 65s most will have some positive radiographic evidence.
- The natural history tends to be one of progression and deterioration, but at unpredictable rates.
- The only 'cure' is by artificial joint replacement. This is feasible and possible for only a few.
- Much relief can be achieved through general measures, drugs and physiotherapy.

CHAPTER 29

RHEUMATOID ARTHRITIS

What is it?

Although joints are the target organs in rheumatoid disease it is a multi-system autoimmune disorder of uncertain cause. It is an ancient condition, having been found in human remains from many centuries past.

The basic pathology is inflammation with tissue destruction and attempts at repair. The rheumatoid factor is present in 80% of those affected.

Females are much more likely to suffer than males (3 : 1) and there seems to be some genetic predisposition. Diagnosis has to be based on clinical features (see page 294) supported by investigations. Although a proportion become severely disabled, the outlook overall in persons seen in general practice is better than hospital experience.

Despite intensive research, the aetiology of RA remains unknown. However, there are three areas which are relevant in the development of RA.

Genetic

Genetic susceptibility has been clearly shown:

- The condition is familial.
- More frequent coincidence in monozygotic than dizygotic twins.
- Associated with the presence of HLA-DR4 in Western Euro-peans – furthermore, the presence of this HLA antigen correlates well with the more serious and complicated forms of the disease.

Autoimmunity

- 80% of patients with RA have auto-antibodies to immuno-globulin G.
- High levels of the antigen, rheumatoid factor, are also associated with the more severe forms of the disease.

Infection

- A variety of organisms have been considered in the aetiology of RA, and discarded for lack of evidence. More recently, viral infections such as rubella and Epstein-Barr infections have been implicated, and further clinical studies are awaited

The fundamental *pathological* change in RA is a chronic non-specific inflammation and proliferation of the synovial membrane. This is followed by destruction of intra-articular cartilage and replacement by pannus. Peri-articular structures such as ligaments and tendons are damaged, and ultimately joint destruction occurs. The final destruction of cartilage, bone, tendons and ligaments probably results from the action of a variety of proteolytic enzymes and other mediators. There may well be an underlying micro-vasculitis also contributing to the destruction of the joint tissues.

Who gets it and when?

The true prevalence is uncertain because diagnosis is imprecise. It is believed that 1–2% of the population have 'active' disease. This means 20–40 persons in a practice of 2000 but in fact only about one-half this number consult their GP annually. It may be that others are labelled as 'arthritis' without the rheumatoid prefix.

Table 29.1 shows the likely annual consulting rates of rheuma-toid arthritis, osteoarthritis and non-specific arthritis in practices of 2000 and 10 000 persons.

TABLE 29.1 Arthritis: annual consultation rates

Disorder	Persons consulting annually	
	per 2000	per 10 000
Rheumatoid arthritis	12	60
Osteoarthritis	48	240
Non-specific 'arthritis'	50	250

Age at onset

Rheumatoid disease can commence at any age but the peak period is in women aged 20–40 (Figure 29.1).

The *age prevalence* based on numbers of persons consulting (Figure 29.2) shows the predominance in women and that its frequency increases with age, but this may be because once started the condition persists for many years.

The *annual incidence* of new cases is 1–2 in a practice of 2000 or 5–10 in a group of 10 000.

Thus in these populations it is likely that during a professional lifetime of 30–40 years a GP will diagnose and manage about 100 patients with rheumatoid disease.

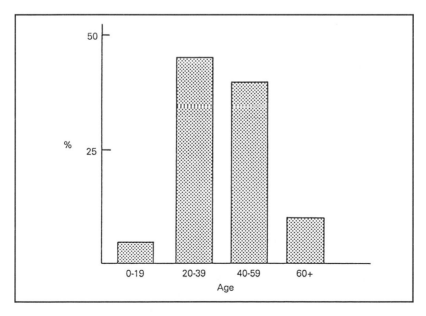

Fig. 29.1—Rheumatoid arthritis – age of onset

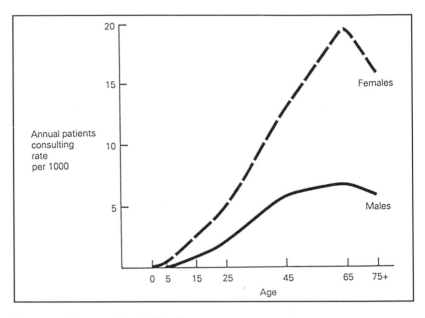

Fig. 29.2—Rheumatoid arthritis – frequency

How does it present?

The *onset* usually is slow and insidious with vague aches and stiffness in affected joints, worse in the morning and easing as the day goes on. On occasions the onset may be acute and dramatic with sweats, high fever and immobility caused by widespread joint involvement.

The *joints affected* are most likely to be hands, with metacarpo-phalangeal joints involved, followed by knees, elbows, shoulders, feet, hips and neck.

There is pain and stiffness accompanied by swelling and limitation of movements.

Systemic disturbance is variable. There is always some feeling of malaise but there also may be sweating, fever, weight loss and anorexia.

Associated diseases: Rheumatoid type arthritis may be a feature of other diseases that should be noted, ie. psoriasis, rubella (transient), diffuse lupus erythematosus, Crohn's disease and Reiter's syndrome.

Complications

Complications may be arthritic and systemic.

Joints may become fixed and deformed. They also may become secondarily infected and be the sites of septic arthritis.

Systemic: Almost any organ may be affected, such as the skin, the central and peripheral nervous system, the eyes, the smaller arteries and veins, the heart and pericardium, the lungs and pleura, the blood (anaemia) and the kidneys (amyloid disease).

Pulmonary complications

Pleural disease

- Common – more in females than males.
- Usually asymptomatic.
- Pleuritic pain with/without effusion can occur; the effusion may need draining if the patient becomes breathless. In up to 20% of patients with effusion, chronic pleural thickening can occur.

Pulmonary nodules

- May involve the pleura or the lung parenchyma, and in this case may mimic lung carcinoma.
- Usually asymptomatic but may become infected leading to cavitation, or sometimes result in rupture into the pleural cavity causing pneumothorax.
- When the nodules are widespread and occur in miners with underlying pneumoconiosis, the condition is called Caplan's syndrome.

Diffuse interstitial fibrosis

Subclinical fibrosis is probably common in RA, since abnormal lung function tests are often seen. It is thought that progression to symptomatic interstitial fibrosis is rare (probably < 1%), and if this does occur treatment with high dose steroids can be tried.

Obliterative bronchiolitis

This is a rare complication and rapidly progressive. It is commoner if other severe systemic complications are present. Steroid treatment is usually unsuccessful and death from respiratory failure is likely to occur within a few months.

Pulmonary amyloidosis

Drug-induced pulmonary damage – gold and penicillamine.

What happens?

As noted, the experience in general practice of the outcome and prognosis is different from that of hospital colleagues. The GP sees all grades, the rheumatologist only those referred by a GP.

Using 4 grades of severity:

---

1. No or minimal disabilities and fully independent.
2. Some disabilities but independent with some aids /appliances.
3. Moderate disabilities – help necessary with daily functions.
4. Severe disabilities – totally dependent on others.

J.F.'s experience of following up rheumatoid patients for 25 years and longer (Table 29.2) shows that moderate–severe disabilities occurred in only one-third of patients and that almost one-half had minimal disabilities.

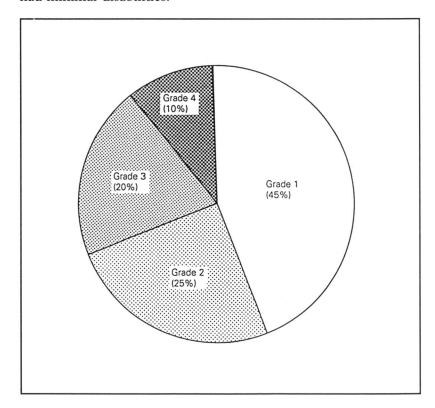

Fig. 29.3—GP experience of rheumatoid patients – grades 1–4 of increasing severity

TABLE 29.2   Rheumatoid arthritis: grades and outcome

Grades	1	2	3	4	Total
%	45	25	20	10	100

In the majority the rheumatoid process appears to subside and if during the period of activity the process is not great then disabilities will not be severe.

Four possible courses are recognized (J.F.):

• Single acute episode affecting one or more joints with full recovery.
• Slow progression but possibility of cessation of activity.
• Progressive deterioration with acute episodes.
• Rapid deterioration, severe illness and disability.

Based on a knowledge of the natural history of the disorder the following points must be noted in order to manage patients effectively:

• Rheumatoid disease has no known *cause* and no specific *cure*.
• The *course* is not necessarily one of progressive deterioration and severe disability – more than one-half will *not* become disabled or dependent.
• Management must aim at controlling the active inflammatory process, maintaining function and hoping for the condition to subside.

What to do?

Assessment

The diagnosis of rheumatoid arthritis must be based on characteristic symptoms and signs supported by some abnormalities on investigation.

Erosive joint changes will be found in radiographs. There may be anaemia. The ESR generally is raised and is a fair measure of the activity of the disease. Abnormal serological rheumatoid factor tests (Rose–Waaler and latex fixation test) will become abnormal in many (4 out of 5) cases.

Assessment of progress is best made on the severity of symptoms and signs and on the functional abilities of patients to carry on with their normal life activities. Results of investigations (ESR and radiography) are less important, though interesting, in continuing assessment.

It may be useful to have all patients assessed initially by a rheumatologist. The advantages of this course are:

- In early cases the diagnosis may be difficult to prove because there may be a normal ESR and no X-ray changes.
- An assessment and explanation of the long-term prognosis given by the rheumatologist might be helpful to the patient.
- The use of drugs such as gold and penicillamine should not necessarily be considered only after non-steroidal anti-inflammatory treatment has failed. Experienced clinical judgement is therefore necessary to decide whether these drugs should be used early on, and this is best done by a rheumatologist.

The subsequent care of the patient is probably best shared between the GP and the rheumatologist.

Aims of treatment

- Relief of current symptoms.
- Prevention of stiffness due to restriction of joint movements.
- Prevent progression and long-term damage to the joints.
- To provide adequate ongoing psychological support in a very depressing and demoralizing disease.

Management

Management can be divided into general care of the patient and the family and social aids; general measures to help the arthritis and disabilities; pain relief; and specific therapy.

The patient and the family should be told of the nature of the condition, its hopeful prognosis (one-half will not be severely disabled), its long duration and the wide scope of treatment.

The *joints* can be helped in many ways. Rest is important in acute stages either by local rest, through splinting or, in general, bed or recumbent rest.

Relief may be obtained through various forms of heat and physiotherapy.

Injections of corticosteroids into affected joints may help but there are risks and dangers – possible secondary infection and increase in joint degeneration.

Pain relief can be obtained through the various analgesics and anti-inflammatory drugs, of which there are many to choose from.

Specific measures through use of gold, anti-immune and cytotoxic drugs or corticosteroids may be considered in progressive and more severe cases.

In severely disorganized joints *surgery* may help through joint replacement or other procedures.

It is always uncertain how much therapy contributes to the ultimate course and outcome of the disease. The natural course is unpredictable at the start. Some may suffer one or two minor episodes and recover completely. Some will continue to suffer minor or moderate attacks with little or some permanent disability. Some, the minority, will progress relentlessly and lead to a state of sever disability and invalidism in spite of all forms of treatment.

Treatment of the acute phase

- Bedrest
- Immobilization of acutely painful joints.
- Relief of pain through heat and physiotherapy.
- *Local intra-articular injection* – if only a single large joint is involved, then it is always worth trying a local injection of hydrocortisone. Sometimes, when relief is obtained it may last for several months without any other treatment being necessary.

Drugs

Aspirin is first choice in the maximum dose tolerated – 4 to 6 grams daily.

NSAIDs – these drugs have little effect on the inflammatory process, but are effective in relieving pain by inhibition of the synthesis of prostaglandins which cause pain and swelling in the joints.

About one-third of patients derive considerable benefit, one-third some relief and one-third fail to respond at all to a NSAID.

It is best to become familiar with just 2 or 3 different drugs; diclonefac (Voltarol) is a good first choice. Tenoxicam (Mobiflex) is suitable for elderly patients since it has a long half-life and can be given once daily. Indomethacin (Indocid) is potent but toxic – gastric irritation, headache, ankle swelling and psychosis can all occur.

It is important to remember that NSAIDs can interact with other drugs and thereby cause problems, e.g. warfarin, tolbutamide, diuretics, antihypertensives and anticonvulsants such as phenytoin.

Long-term treatment of RA

General measures

- Education on nature of RA, prognosis, benefits and limitations of available treatment.
- Look for and treat iron-deficiency anaemia due to chronic blood loss from treatment with aspirin or NSAIDs.
- Psychological support and treatment of depression.

Physiotherapy

This can be as beneficial as drug treatment in appropriate patients:

- Exercise programmes
- Rest splints especially for wrists
- Physiotherapy and hydrotherapy for increasing mobility
- Chiropody and attention to footwear.

Drug treatment

NSAIDs can be tried first and, if successful, continued until symptoms have been fully relieved. After symptoms have been controlled for several weeks, it is worth trying to reduce the dose, and, if possible, stop the drug altogether. A further course of treatment can then be given if the RA flares up again.

Slow-acting drugs for RA:

These include gold, sulphasalazine, penicillamine, azathioprine, methotrexate and chloroquine. These drugs do reduce inflammation in the joints, unlike NSAIDs, and take one to three months to attain their full effect.

Indications: They are the next choice if NSAIDs are ineffective, but their use should not be limited to when the NSAIDs have failed. Since there is some evidence that some of these drugs, e.g. gold and sulphasalazine, may be able to prevent long-term damage to the joints, it is worth considering their early use if progressive joint damage is envisaged, e.g. in a particularly severe form of the disease with systemic complications.

The *duration of use* of these drugs is not known, and some patients may need to continue them for many years to keep the condition under adequate control.

Choice of drug: They are probably all equally effective, and the choice of a particular drug may well be based on its tolerability and side-effects. Gold is probably most often the first choice.

Gold – the main limitation to use has been the need for injections every one or two weeks. Side-effects are rashes, glomerular damage and depression of the white cell count; mouth ulcers and colitis can also be a problem. The white cell count shold be monitored regularly.

Sulphasalazine – is increasingly used since it has few side-effects and is effective in seronegative disease (no rheumatoid factor in the blood) as well as seropositive disease. It is perhaps the treatment of choice for the GP in resistant patients. The course of treatment should be restricted initially to 3 months:

- one third derive major benefit
- one third derive some benefit
- one third derive no relief.

The side-effects include nausea or vomiting, occasional neutropenia and a reversible depression of the sperm count.

Penicillamine – is given orally and results in improvement in 50–60% of patients. It is not used so frequently now because of the efficacy and relative safety of sulphasalazine. Side-effects includes rashes, loss of taste, vomiting, mouth ulcers, renal damage and pancytopenia.

Other drugs which may be used in difficult cases include chloroquine (there is a risk of retinal damage), azathioprine (minimal risk of bone marrow oncogenicity) and methotrexate (risk of liver and bone-marrow toxicity).

Long-term steroids in RA:

Steroids are indicated if there are life-threatening complications of RA such as severe vasculitis but their long-term toxicity is otherwise unacceptable in treating what can be a very chronic disease; this applies especially to young patients with RA.

Steroids may be of value in the elderly if used in small doses (2.5–5.0 mg/day) when the RA is severe and unresponsive to other measures.

One way in which steroid treatment may be useful and safe is by occasional booster injections of 125 mg of prednisolone acetate in patients on a very low dose of 1 mg daily maintenance treatment.

Indications for surgery in RA

- Severe unremitting pain unresponsive to medical treatment.
- Progressive deterioration of joint function.
- Severe joint instability.
- Unacceptable loss of joint mobility.

- Progressive joint destruction on X-ray.
- Surgical complications:
  tendon rupture
  carpal tunnel syndrome
  severe ankle disease
  resistant synovitis in a single joint.

Practical points

- Rheumatoid disease involves more than joints; it is probably a systemic autoimmune disorder with joints and lungs being most affected.
- Onset at any age but most often at 20–40. Females outnumber males by 3 : 1.
- A GP with 2000 patients can expect 1–2 new cases annually and a further 12 who will consult.
- Prognosis is not uniformly bad – only 30% will become severely disabled.
- General advice, support and provision of home assistance and aids are important.
- It may be helpful to refer the patient to a rheumatologist for an initial assessment and discussion.
- Physical treatment can be as effective as drugs in some patients.
- Intra-articular injection of hydrocortisone is always worth considering if a single joint is affected; otherwise, aspirin is probably the best drug to use for the initial treatment of an acute flare-up of RA.
- Most of the NSAIDs have similar efficacy; therefore the choice of drug should be based on its tolerability and side-effects.
- NSAIDs do not reduce joint inflammation, but the slow-acting drugs, like gold and sulphasalazine, do. These drugs may therefore be the treatment of choice where progressive joint damage is envisaged, e.g. in severe RA, and their use should not be reserved for NSAID failure only.
- Long-term steroid treatment should only be used if life-threatening complications are present, e.g. severe vasculitis, and all other treatment has failed.

CHAPTER **30**

NON-ARTICULAR AND OTHER FORMS OF RHEUMATISM

What are they?

Almost one-third of all persons consulting for musculo-skeletal disorders do so for rather non-specific conditions, such as:

- tendinitis
- bursitis
- shoulder capsulitis and frozen shoulder
- fibrositis
- polymyalgia
- gout
- other aches and pains in limbs.

It is believed that they represent inflammatory reactions possibly resulting from overuse, misuse, trauma or for no known reason.

Who gets them and when?

The numbers of persons consulting annually for these conditions is shown in Table 30.1.

TABLE 30.1 Annual consultation rates for non-articular and other forms of rheumatism

Disorder	Persons consulting annually	
	per 2000	per 10 000
Tendinitis	24	120
Bursitis	10	50
Shoulder lesions	14	70
'Fibrositis'	25	125
Polymyalgia	1	5
Gout	6	30
Others	20	100
Total	100	500

The *age distribution* of most of these conditions (Figure 30.1) includes adults of all ages but with a peak at 45–65. Polymyalgia is rare below the age of 65.

Males suffer more from knee problems and gout, *females* more from all other types.

How do they present?

The common feature is pain and tenderness local to the affected part and also painful limitation of movements.

Some particular syndromes:

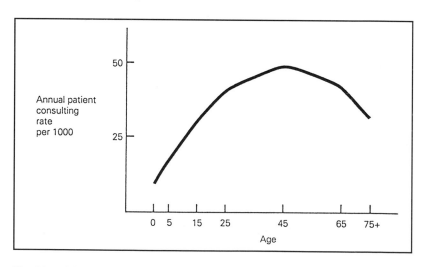

Fig. 30.1—Non-articular rheumatism – age prevalence

- *Tennis elbow/golfer's elbow* are epicaudylitis of lateral or medial parts of the elbows respectively.
- *De Quervain's syndrome* is a local tendinitis of extensor tendons of thumb at wrist.
- *Creaking tenosynovitis of the forearm extensors* causes pain during movements and characteristic crepitus (best heard with stethoscope, or felt).
- *Shoulder pains* are difficult to specify but supraspinatus tendinitia has localized tenderness and pain on abduction of shoulder; 'frozen shoulder' produces considerable pain and stiffness in all directions.
- *Bursitis* can occur in various sites such as knees, hips, ankles, elbows, shoulders and hallux with painful swellings.
- *'Fibrositis'* is a hypothetical term for areas of muscular pain and tenderness in back and neck areas and around shoulders and hips.
- *Polymyalgia* occurs in elderly persons with severe pain and muscle stiffness (worse in mornings) accompanied by considerable malaise and distress, characterized by a very high ESR, often over 100 mm per hour. It may also be associated with temporal arteritis. Apart from high ESR its diagnosis can be supported by dramatic and rapid improvement on taking oral steroids.
- *Gout* classically affects men with an acute arthritis of first metatarso phalangeal joints, but it can also cause pain in soft tissues. More common recently in women as well as men because of blood uricaemia secondary to medication with diuretics (see pages 169).

What happens?

All these conditions, apart from polymyalgia and gout, tend to improve and clear naturally, given time. It may take a few days, weeks or even months (in frozen shoulder).

What to do?

Assessment

Although these rather non-specific conditions are common and resolve and respond to simple measures it must be realized that similar aches and pains may be the early symptoms of serious disorders such as:

- rheumatoid and similar inflammatory conditions;

- neoplastic diseases such as secondary bone deposits and primary myelomatosis.

In most instances investigations are not necessary but an ESR and/or local straight X-rays may be indicated.

Management

Although spontaneous resolution is likely, it may be a long time coming, and relief is important.

As a first line, simple analgesics or NSAIDs in adequate doses should be prescribed.

However, the most effective and rapid treatment is local injection of a steroid preparation into the most tender site, usually with a local anaesthetic. Pain may be aggravated for a day or two but then complete or almost complete relief is likely. Repeat injections may be required monthly for a few months.

Various physiotherapeutic measures may help but it is difficult to select these cases.

Practical points

- Non-articular soft tissue disorders are the largest group of rheumatic disorders.
- Included are tendinitis, bursitis, capsulitis and fibrositis – more rarely polymyalgia and non-articular gout.
- Peak prevalence is at ages 45–65 and most will resolve naturally in a few weeks.
- Rapid relief usually follows local injection of a steroid preparation.
- Beware of the rare possibility of serious disorders such as malignancies presenting as vague aches and pains.

SECTION VI

OBSTETRICS, GYNAECOLOGY AND UROLOGY

CHAPTER 31

OBSTETRICS AND GYNAECOLOGY (OBG) – THE CLINICAL SPECTRUM

OBG is a major part of general practice in the UK. The general practitioner is involved in family planning, antenatal and postnatal care, all types of gynaecological problems, preventive care through cervical smears, and in general advice on normal and abnormal marital and sexual matters.

Obstetrics

The *annual birth rate* in the UK at present is 14 per 1000; this means 28 per GP with 2000 patients, or 140 per group with 10 000 (Table 31.1).

The *fertility rate*, i.e. number of children per woman (or couple), is now 1.8, which means that the population would be likely to fall without immigration.

Almost all practices now are involved in providing *antenatal care*, shared with local specialist-hospital services, to all pregnant women.

TABLE 31.1 Annual pregnancies and outcomes

	Annual pregnancies	
	per 2000	per 10 000
Total conceptions	38	190
Births		
Natural	22	110
Assisted	3	15
Caesarean section	3	15
Total	28	140
Abortions		
Spontaneous	5	20
Terminations	5	20
Ectopic pregnancy	1 in 2 years	2–3
Infant mortality	1 in 5 years	Less than 1
Maternal mortality	1 in 400 years	1 in 80 years
Major congenital birth defect	1 in 8 years	Less than 1
Place of birth		
Hospital	99%	99%
Shared AN care		
GP and hospital	85%	100%

In addition, in a practice population of 2000, there will be annually:

- 5 natural *spontaneous abortions*
- 5 *legal terminations of pregnancy* (TOP) (two in NHS hospitals and three in private clinics)
- an *ectopic pregnancy* is likely to occur every 2 years.

Place of delivery

99% of deliveries now take place in hospital. GPs are involved in less than 1 in 5 of all deliveries.

Outcome of pregnancy

- In 70% the *antenatal period* is normal, in the others the most likely abnormalities are raised blood pressure and toxaemia.
- In 80% the *delivery* is spontaneous and natural.
- In 10% it is assisted by forceps or vacuum extractor.
- In 10% a Caesarean section is performed.
- *Infant mortality rate* is now under 10 per 1000 births.

- *Maternal mortality rate* is now under 1 per 10 000 births.
- Significant *congenital abnormalities* in the baby occur in 5 per 1000 births.

Implications

Each GP can expect 28 births annually in his practice. Of these, 22 will be natural deliveries and 6 complicated.

With such small numbers, the continuing experience of a GP in abnormal obstetrics (deliveries) will be minimal.

It is also generally accepted that midwives are best to supervise normal deliveries.

Providing that abnormal deliveries can be anticipated and referred, then home deliveries may be acceptable risks.

Gynaecology

Gynaecological problems make up 10% of all consultations in general practice.

20% of all women consult annually for gynaecological conditions – the proportion is 1 in 3 for the 20–60 age group.

Table 31.2 shows the numbers of women consulting in a year for specific disorders.

TABLE 31.2 Annual consultation rates for gynaecological disorders

	Women consulting annually	
	per 2000	per 10 000
Breast conditions	15	75
Menstrual problems	75	375
Premenstrual tension	20	100
Menopausal disorders	30	150
Vaginitis	20	100
Cervicitis and erosion	3	15
Fibroids	3	15
Ovarian cyst	less than 1	4–5
Prolapse (vaginal)	5	25
Pelvic inflammatory disease	3	15
Sterility	5	25
Cancers	2	10
Breast (new)	1	5
Ovary (new)	1 in 5 years	1
Cervix (new)	1 in 6 years	less than 1
Uterus body (new)	1 in 7 years	less than 1
Others	18	90

The age prevalence is shown in Figure 31.1.

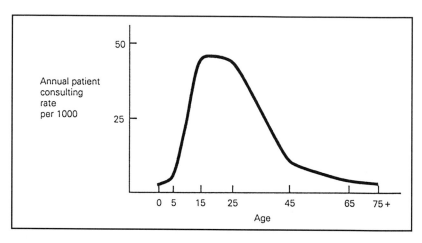

Fig. 31.1—Prevalence of gynaecological problems (RCGP/OPCS, 1986)

Hospital admissions

A GP with 2000 patients can expect to refer 35 patients for hospital admission in a year:

- D and C   5
- hysterectomy   3
- prolapse repair   2
- oviduct operation   2
- cancers   2
- T.O.P.
      (termination of pregnancy)   5 (3 in non-NHS clinics)
- spontaneous abortion   3
- colposcopy, etc.   5
- laparoscopy   5
- others   3

Prevention

Family planning and cervical smears are sizable components of general practice.

In a year, a GP with 2000 patients can expect:

- 60 women for family planning

- 140 women for cervical smears (about 1 in 5 of these will need to be repeated)

Deaths

The major causes of death are cancers.

Annual deaths from:

- cancer of breast   15 000
- ovarian cancer   4 500
- cervical cancer   2 000
- uterine body cancer   1 500

- Total   23 000

In addition, another 500 women die annually from other gynaecological diseases.

Gynaecology – common diseases

Breast disorders

Cancer of the breast is a fear that all women have. Fortunately it is uncommon. More prevalent are benign conditions.

Table 31.3 shows the annual numbers of women likely to be seen in a year in a practice of 2000.

TABLE 31.3 Annual consultation rates for breast disorders in a practice of 2000

Breast cancer	
new case	1
old cases (follow up)	4
Fibrocystic disorders	3
Fibroadenomata	1
Painful breasts	4
Large–small breasts	2

Women come for reassurance and advice. Reassurance that they do not have cancer and advice on what to do for their problems.

If a *lump or swelling* is detected, then referral to a specialist is essential to establish a diagnosis. No woman should have an undiagnosed lump in her breast.

If a breast cyst is suspected, then it is justifiable to attempt to aspirate it and reassure the patient, but follow-up is necessary.

Painful breasts, usually related to the menstrual cycle, are common and the majority of women do not attend for consultation. Relief is not easy. If taking a contraceptive pill, this should be stopped or changed. If explanation does not relieve and reassure, then consideration for medication with tamoxifen or bromocriptine may be advisable, preferably with specialist advice.

Large–small breasts: women may be extremely sensitive and distressed, their feelings must be taken seriously, and the question of plastic procedures discussed fully prior to referral to specialist.

Menstrual problems

Excessive, irregular, scanty or missed *menses* are a common reason for consultation.

First consideration must be to decide whether the condition is *'physiological'*, a variant of normal, or *'pathological'*, resulting from an underlying disorder such as pregnancy, fibroids, neoplasia or hormonal imbalance.

If pathological conditions are excluded, then the temptation to treat speculatively with various hormones should be resisted.

Note the possibility of a secondary anaemia with heavy menses – sometimes correcting this with oral iron helps the heavy menses.

Premenstrual tension – mood changes, painful breasts, bloating and weight gain, headaches and other symptoms are parts of this common syndrome.

The multiplicity of recommended treatments with hormones, diuretics, psychotropics and other substances implies that there is no reliable method of relief.

Explanation and support are most important even if other methods are tried.

Menopausal symptoms

These affect the majority of women, but relatively few seek medical advice.

The question of whether to prescribe hormone replacement therapy (HRT) is a debatable one; secondly, should it be short-term or long-term prophylactic management to prevent possible osteoporosis?

At present short-term HRT is more popular than long-term because of uncertainties over side-effects as well as benefits.

Infections

Vaginal discharge is very common. In the majority it is a *physiological* excess of normal secretions, but *pathological* infective and other causes must be excluded.

Possible specific infections are chlamydia, candida, trichomonas and gardnerella. Gonococcal infections are much less frequent. If detected on investigation, then specific treatment must be given.

Chronic cervicitis, endometrial polyps and, of course, cancers of cervix and uterus are possible, but more unlikely causes of discharge.

Pelvic inflammatory disease is less common but more serious and difficult to treat. Serious because of the immediate effects with pain and possible intra-abdominal complications, but also because of possible sterility. The conditions are not easy to diagnose — particularly the subacute and chronic types. Nor is treatment with antibiotics completely effective.

Contraception

At any time 3 out of 4 women in the reproductive age groups use some forms of contraception:

• Pill	20%
• Condom	25%
• I.U.D.	10%
• Diaphragm	10%
• Other methods	10%

The GP or family planning clinic will be consulted for prescriptions for the contraceptive pill, diaphragm or I.U.D.

Cervical cytology

It is government policy that all women between 25–65 should have a cervical smear as a preventive measure for early diagnosis of cervical cancer and a GP with 2000 patients (or the practice nurse) can expect to carry out 140 such procedures each year.

Unfortunately the benefits of these procedures are uncertain since the annual mortality from cervical cancer has remained around 2000 deaths for the past 20 years.

Some UK national facts should be noted:

Annual numbers for UK

Cervical smears	5 million
'Abnormal smears'	500 000
Cancer of cervix registered	4 000
Deaths from cervical cancer	2 000

Cancers

To keep numbers in perspective, it is useful to remember that in a practice of 2000 persons the likely rates for new gynaecological cancers will be:

- Breast   1 new case per year
- Ovary   1 new case every 5 years
- Cervix   1 new case every 6 years
- Body of uterus 1 new case every 7 years

CHAPTER 32

URINARY TRACT DISEASES – THE CLINICAL SPECTRUM

Urological disorders are uncommon, apart from acute infections in women. The 'specialist' diseases so common in hospital practice are infrequent in general practice. Thus, a group with 10 000 patients may have one patient with chronic renal failure and perhaps two who have had kidney transplants. A kidney tumour can be expected once every 10 years by a GP with 2000 patients, and a testicular neoplasm once every 15 years.

However, now cases of prostatic cancer and bladder cancer will each occur once a year.

Patient consulting rates

In a year, only 4% of patients listed consult for urinary tract disorders. Of these (Table 32.1), more than one-half will be acute urinary tract infections in women (see Chapter 33).

The other group of note are the various male genital conditions.

317

Hospital admissions

5% of hospital admissions are for urological disorders with cysto-scopy, prostatectomy and circumcision being the main groups.

TABLE 32.1   Annual patient consulting rates for urinary tract disorders

Disease	Patients consulting annually	
	per 2000	per 10 000
Acute infections		
Cystitis	45	225
Pyelitis	5	25
Total	50	250
Renal calculi	4	20
Chronic renal failure	1	5
Neoplasms	2	10
Male genital		
Enlarged prostate	8	40
Hydrocele	2	10
Epididymo-orchitis	2	10
Balanitis	8	40
Other male disorders	6	30
Total	26	130
Others	6	30

(*Source*: Third Morbidity Survey)

Causes of death

Only 3% of deaths are from urological disorders, most from neoplasms.

CHAPTER 33

ACUTE URINARY INFECTIONS

What are they?

Infections of the urinary tract are common. They occur in practice at an annual prevalence rate or 25 per 1000.

Although they are so frequent there is still much uncertainty and much controversy over their nature, outcome and significance and therefore of their management.

The urinary tract is particularly liable to infection with *Escherichia coli* (*E. coli*) bacteria, although other organisms such as tubercle bacilli, pseudomonas and a few others can also cause recognizable infections.

The infecting strains of *E. coli* are similar to those found in faeces and therefore it is likely that the source of infection is from the large gut.

Urinary infections are much more prevalent in women than in men, particularly in young women, and this suggests that the infection is an ascending one through the shorter female urethra and associated with active sexual behaviour.

Bloodstream infection is possible also and is the likely route in tuberculosis of the urinary tract.

There are a number of groups specially vulnerable to urinary infections: women in the reproductive period at 20–50 years, women during pregnancy, the aged of both sexes, and young girls.

In most urinary infections there is no obvious underlying abnormality of the urinary tract but the most dangerous types of urinary infections are those secondary to congenital abnormalities, those with obstruction to urinary flow, with neoplasms or calculi and those associated with neurological diseases affecting bladder function.

There is poor correlation between clinical symptoms and signs and those investigations carried out to define the site and pathology of the condition.

Particularly important are urinary infections in young children with urinary reflux from the bladder into the ureters, with subacute or silent infection, and dangers of renal scarring and loss of function.

Some infections of the urinary tract may be 'silent' with no urinary symptoms but with possibly dangerous and serious effects from renal damage and failure.

Causal organisms can be detected from only about one-half of those with symptoms, but in the others, with similar symptoms of frequency and dysuria, no organisms can be found in the urines.

Clinical symptoms and signs may not be helpful in separating acute cystitis, acute pyelitis or acute urethritis.

Attempts have been made to detect 'silent' infections by screening urines of apparently normal persons for bacteriuria and picking out those with more than 100000 organisms per ml for further investigations as potentially infected subjects.

Such screening exercises have shown an increase with age from a low rate of 0.2% of bacteriuria in boys and 1% in girls to a high of 25% in 80-year-old men and women. The true significance of bacteriuria in the absence of symptoms is not known and it would be wrong to assume that it indicates a possible serious outcome in all cases, but it is of importance in early pregnancy.

The most important consideration in dealing with acute urinary infections is to achieve some effective working clinical philosophy. Should they be considered as minor and frequent annoyances and treated in an *ad hoc* fashion with anti-bacterial drugs as and when they occur, or should they be taken much more seriously and each case investigated fully in order to treat energetically and prevent the long-term development of chronic pyelonephritis, renal failure and death? These are extreme views and the best approach lies between them requiring skill, judgment, experience and art as well as science for good care.

Who gets them when?

In a practice of 2000, 50 persons will consult annually for acute urinary tract infections. The female : male ratio is 5 : 1. Figure 33.1 shows the *age and sex prevalence rates*:

- prevalence higher in females except in elderly
- not shown – more male infants (neonates) have congenital urinary tract abnormalities and likely infections – but numbers are very small
- in females highest prevalence is in reproductive age group 20–50
- high rates (not shown) during pregnancy.

How do they present?

Although the most usual clinical presentation is with frequency and dysuria and variable degrees of general malaise, there are other forms.

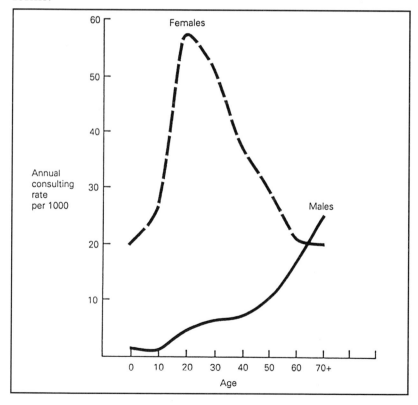

Fig. 33.1—Acute urinary infection – annual consulting rates

To relate these to diagnostic labels:

- *Cystitis* is the most prevalent type especially in women with sudden dysuria, frequency, lower abdominal ache and backache, but with no great general ill health.
- *Pyelitis* is much less frequent. The main feature is that of an acute systemic infection with fever, rigors, ache and sweats, pain in loin with tenderness and frequency and dysuria being less prominent symptoms.
- *Chronic renal failure* is a very rare end result of urinary infections.

Different clinical patterns occur at different ages

In *children* acute urinary infections may be silent and insidious and present as slow and retarded physical development or non-thriving in infants and general poor health.

The attacks may also be violent and explosive with high fever, convulsions, vomiting and abdominal pain, yet with few or no localizing urinary symptoms. 'PUO' (pyrexia of unknown origin) may be caused by an underlying smouldering urinary infection.

Most often acute urinary infections in childhood occur in little girls with dysuria, frequency and some abdominal pain, and are easy to recognize.

Most enuretics have a normal and uninfected urinary tract, but in a few enuresis may be a feature of urinary infection.

In *adult females* (20–50) acute urinary infections are common.

Most present as 'acute cystitis' with sudden frequency and dysuria. Haematuria may occur. The urine has an unpleasant fishy smell. Fever, rigors and backache are unusual and when present the diagnosis of 'acute pyelitis' is made.

During *pregnancy* bacteriuria is found in 5–10% of all women. This group is more likely than others to develop pyelitis during pregnancy. Some 20% of these bacteriurics do develop clinical acute urinary infections. However, this represents a rate of only 1–2% in all pregnancies.

With *increasing age* acute urinary infections tend to present as frequency and/or dysuria, particularly in men, or more silently in elderly women. In men the underlying cause is most often enlargement of the prostate and in women an atony of the bladder with some bladder neck obstruction and perhaps associated uterine prolapse with a cystocoele.

What happens?

As noted the most likely ages of onset of first attacks of acute urinary infections are between 20 and 40 years of age in women and over the age of 60 in men.

Once a person has suffered from an attack of acute urinary infection, recurrences are likely in 40% of women and in 15% of men.

There is a small group of women, between 20 and 50, who suffer numerous attacks annually.

The outcome in persons with acute urinary infections depends on any underlying serious cause. It will be less satisfactory in persons with congenital or other structural abnormalities of the urinary tract, than in those in whom no abnormalities are detected on investigation.

Taking all persons who present with acute urinary infections, an important cause is found in 10%. Such underlying primary causes are more likely in affected males at all ages, in those with clinical features of an upper urinary infection (pyelitis), in those with recurrent attacks, and in those who have some unusual accompanying clinical features such as haematuria or renal colic.

In the majority of persons with acute urinary infections in whom no serious underlying cause is present the natural history is a tendency for attacks to cease in time, without any evidence of permanent serious renal damage (Figure 33.2). Even those who go through a phase of frequent attacks eventually cease to suffer attacks.

Chronic renal failure is rarely related clinically with a history of recurrent or persistent urinary infections. In GP experience (J.F.) the rate of new cases of chronic renal failure has been 1 every 5 years, compared with the 50 annual cases of acute infections.

Another feature is that males are as likely to suffer renal failure as females, again contrary to the common acute infections.

What to do?

Assessment

A step by step procedure:

(1) *Is it an acute urinary infection?*

Acute urinary infections are frequent. They are easy to diagnose when clinical features point to the urinary tract, but their possibility must be remembered in any acute fever and in cases of general ill health.

The diagnosis of a urinary infection cannot be made without testing the urine.

(2) Further investigations?

Most common acute urinary infections in women do not require special investigations. It is reasonable to assume, at first, that they are suffering from a benign and self-limiting condition.

Further investigations are indicated in the following circumstances:

- Recurrent attacks in all persons.
- Children should be further investigated to exclude possible remediable congenital defects, e.g. vesico-ureteric reflux.
- It is stated that boys should all be investigated following any acute urinary infection but that girls need not be investigated unless they suffer recurrent attacks. It is wiser to investigate all children who suffer an acute urinary infection.
- All men who have suffered an attack of acute urinary infection should be further investigated.
- All who have suffered from an acute pyelitis should be further investigated.
- The situation is more difficult in the elderly. Certainly those with recurrent clinical attacks should be investigated and, in particular, men who have prostatic symptoms.

The further investigations might be ultrasound, intravenous urography and tests of renal function.

Cystoscopy should be carried out to exclude bladder or bladder neck pathology.

(3) Referral to a specialist

Most cases of acute urinary infections can be investigated by the family physician in the first instance.

Referral to a specialist must follow when an underlying condition requiring further surgical or medical care is discovered or is suspected or when recurrent attacks continue, or when there is no response to treatment.

The majority of acute urinary infections can be treated outside hospital, unless the course is unusual.

(4) Screening for bacteriuria

Wholesale population screening for bacteriuria has no sound basis except in children and pregnant women.

Management

Those with attacks of acute urinary infection can and do recover, untreated, spontaneously without the physician ever being consulted.

It is unknown exactly what proportion of all urinary infections are ever taken to the physician. Since the prevalence of bacteriuria in the population is about 5% and since the annual prevalence of clinical acute urinary infections is 1.5% there must be many bacteriurics who are untreated and untroubled.

When the patient with an acute urinary infection does present to the physician and a diagnosis has been made, the management is three-fold:

- immediate treatment
- follow-up and investigation
- long-term care and prevention.

Immediate treatment

In one-half of those with symptoms of acute urinary infection who are investigated, no pathogenic organism will be detected. *E. coli* is the organism detected most often.

It cannot be assumed that those cases in which no pathogens are isolated are due to viruses or some other organisms. It is more likely that our methods of investigation may be less than completely reliable. As a therapeutic assumption for immediate action it is justifiable to assume that the most likely pathogen is *E. coli*.

There is a wide choice of antibiotic and antibacterial drugs, such as:

- ampicillin
- amoxycillin
- cotrimoxazole
- trimethoprim
- nitrofurantoin and cephalosporins

Whichever one is chosen it should be given in adequate dosage and duration to achieve control of infection.

Follow-up and investigation

Patients treated for urinary infections should be followed up until the urine becomes clear of infection and symptoms are relieved.

Bacteriological examination of the urine to check recovery should be carried out 2–4 weeks from onset. This allows time for recovery and avoids over-frequent and unnecessary investigations.

If the urine is clear of infection and the patient is well, no further action need be taken. However, if the urine is infected and in recurrences, further investigations should be undertaken.

Long-term care and prevention

A small group of women are liable to recurrent attacks of cystitis and a smaller group of persons with persistent infection require long-term care and supervision. They may need personal advice on possible preventive measures, long-term prophylactic chemotherapy, or surgical procedures to correct structural abnormalities.

Practical points

- Acute urinary infections are frequent: 50 per year in a practice of 2000.
- Those most liable to attacks are women between 20 and 50, the elderly and young girls.
- The natural history in women with cystitis is for onset at 20–40 years, some recurrences, and then for the attacks to cease after 50 years of age. The outcome is satisfactory without any permanent renal damage.
- Infections may be associated with some underlying abnormalities in the urinary tract such as congenital lesions, calculi, neoplasms, or obstructions at the bladder neck or at other sites.
- Chronic pyelonephritis is a rare condition with a likely annual incidence of less than 0.1 per 1000.
- In assessment, the questions that have to be answered are: Is there urinary infection present? What further investigations are necessary? Is referral to a specialist necessary?
- Management of the acute attack should be to control the immediate infection, to follow up and ensure recovery and clearing of the infection, to investigate certain groups and to organize long-term care of those with persistent infections.

SECTION VII

PSYCHIATRY

CHAPTER 34

PSYCHIATRIC DISORDERS – THE CLINICAL SPECTRUM

The first shock and rude awakening that affects the physician on entering the field of primary care practice is a mass of apparently unrecognized, undefinable and unfamiliar emotional disorders.

In his training in the seclusion of medical school and hospitals he had been sheltered and protected from the fact that many persons find their life situations and circumstances difficult, trying, boring and unsatisfactory, and that they react and rebel with nervous and emotional reactions.

It is when he enters practice and begins to treat people that the young physician begins to appreciate the importance of relating management to the patient, his personality and temperament, family and genetic and social background; to the disease and the GP's own understanding of its nature, course and outcome; and to his own interests, skills and readiness to become involved in good care for his patients.

The second shock comes with the realization that 'cure' is rarely achievable with these conditions and it should not be the overall objective.

Emotional disorders are often the individual's expression of stress and ennui. They form part of that individual's make-up and their appearance and occurrence are likely throughout a lifetime.

'Cure' or recovery from an episode of emotional disorder is satisfying but it should not be a surprise or a disappointment if the condition should recur at sometime. Recurrences are merely a part of the individual's make-up. Once the physician accepts the fact that cure is not a reality and that relief, comfort and support over a lifetime are necessary, then management and relations become easier and results of care better.

The third shock facing the scientifically and academically trained modern physician is the realization that emotional disorders cannot be categorized neatly or labelled or diagnosed with any accuracy or on objective bases.

Syndromes emerge from within the mass of emotional disorders but they are imprecise and become more important to the individual physician in helping him to understand the course and management.

In considering what are the emotional disorders it is necessary, of course, to try to pick out those syndromes which have been well described such as schizophrenia, dementia, mental deficiency and other major psychoses, but these represent only a small proportion of the common mass of such disorders facing the practising primary physician. The great majority are the anxieties, depressions, personality problems, tension, grief and general unhappiness, dissatisfaction and reactions to life and its problems.

The most practical approach is for the individual physician to build up his own understanding, philosophy and approach to the common mass of emotional problems, based on experience supported by data and facts.

Patient consulting rates

In my practice (J.F.) up to 15% of patients consult once or more times each year with some diagnosis of a psychiatric problem. This means 300 in a practice of 2000.

Table 34.1 shows the numbers of persons with various diagnoses, accepting that one person may have more than one diagnosis.

Note that *depression and anxiety* make up two-thirds of all psychiatric diagnoses. It is likely that the number of persons with *alcohol-related problems* is higher than the number who consult.

Although *dementia* is emphasized as an increasing problem, a GP with 2000 persons will have only 10 in his practice and most of these are relatively mild. Only two or so are likely to cause major problems.

TABLE 34.1   Annual consultation rates for psychiatric problems

Diagnosis	Persons consulting annually	
	per 2000	per 10 000
Depression	120	600
Anxiety	80	400
'Stress'	20	100
Psychosomatic	20	100
Child behaviour	5	25
Alcohol–drug dependency	10	50
Phobias	10	50
Dementia – presenile and senile	10	50
Schizophrenia	3	15
Manic-depression	2	10
Parasuicide	3	15
Suicide	1 in 7 years	less than 1
Others	17	65

Schizophrenia and manic-depression are uncommon as is *suicide*. The number of children with '*behaviour problems*' is likely to be an underestimate.

Grades of illness

As with other conditions the majority of the psychiatric disorders seen in general practice are mild but one-third are likely to be chronic (recurrent or persistent) and only 1 in 10 serious.

Grades of illness of psychiatric disorders

minor	55%
chronic	35%
major	10%

Age–sex prevalence

Twice as many females as males consult for psychiatric problems.

The *age prevalence* (Figure 34.1) shows peak consultations at ages 25–55 but also appreciable rates in the elderly.

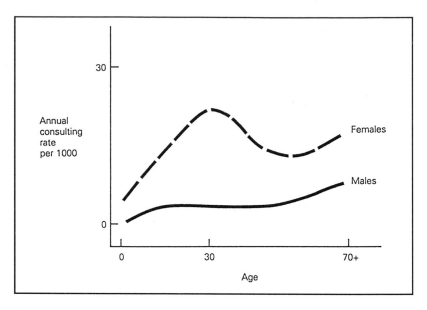

Fig. 34.1—Age prevalence of psychiatric disorders

Sickness-invalidity

14% of all certified sickness absence from work is due to psychiatric problems.

Hospital referrals

Less than 1 in 10 of persons who consult their GP with a psychiatric diagnosis is referred to a psychiatrist.

Some 10 persons in a practice of 2000 will be in hospital with psychiatric disorders each year – three parasuicides, two long-term and five in and out.

Deaths

There are 4500 suicides per year in the UK or one every 7 years in a practice of 2000.

Practical points

- 15% of patients consult in a year for some psychiatric problem.
- Present as a confusing mass of symptoms, often indefinable and difficult to label.
- Depression (120 patients in a practice of 2000) and anxiety (80) are the most frequent groups – often difficult to separate.
- Psychoses are uncommon, five patients per year.
- Suicide only once in 7 years but three parasuicides per year.
- Most (55%) of these problems that present to a GP are minor, 35% are chronic and 10% major.
- Occur at all ages with peak prevalence in women at ages 25–55.
- Only 1 in 10 of those seen will be referred to a psychiatrist.

CHAPTER 35

DEPRESSION

What is it?

From within the mass of emotional disorders the state of depression can be separated. This is a condition of subjective mood accompanied by various somatic symptoms. It is an important condition because it may have some causal basis of disordered metabolism, for which effective antidepressant drugs are available. It is important also in that up to 4500 suicides occur each year in Britain out of more than 100 000 gestures or attempts, which might be preventable.

Who gets it when?

Because of the lack of precision in diagnosis it is difficult to give accurate data on the frequency of depression in the community.

The annual prevalence by patients consulting is 120 per 2000. This represents only about one-quarter of those who are depressed; others do not seek medical advice. Therefore the true prevalence is almost 500 persons per GP.

Only 1 in 10 of those who consult is referred to a psychiatrist.

Suicide is a risk in depression. Its frequency and that of suicide attempts (parasuicide) are shown in Figure 35.1. It is suggested that the annual rate for attempted suicides is under 2 per 1000 of the population and the actual suicide rate is 0.1 per 1000.

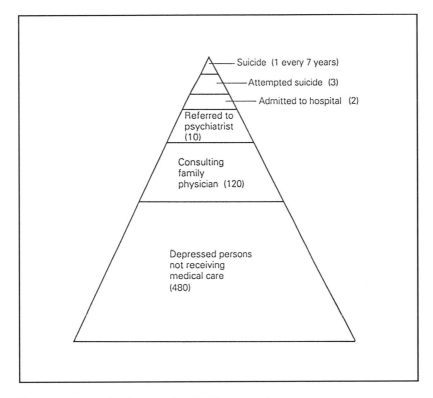

Fig. 35.1—Depression in a practice (2000) community

This means that in an average practice of 2000 there are

- 480 depressed persons
- 120 will consult the practitioner annually
- 3 suicide attempts made each year
- A suicide will occur once every 7 years.

How does it present?

Depression is one of the most overlooked of conditions, with a protean presentation.

It may present with a prominent mood of depression but it may present also in a masked form under the guise of all sorts of quasi-physical symptoms.

The first rule in sound management of depression is to be aware of its possibility. With better and more specific drugs available, the diagnosis of depression is being made more often than in the past and the label of 'depression' is tending to displace others such as 'anxiety', 'neurasthenia' or 'nervous debility'.

Striking symptoms of depression are loss of energy and loss of interest. Requests for 'tonics' and complaints of 'tiredness' are features of depression. The patients feel weak and unwell but find it difficult to formulate their story. They are reticent and disinclined to seek medical advice and help. This reticence is the result of a combination of the depression itself with the vagueness of symptoms and inability of the patients to translate their feelings into medical language. In attempts to fit medical nomenclature, depressed patients may relate their symptoms to overwork, prolonged 'flu', effects of a minor accident or some other recent, or not so recent, personal happening.

Sleep disturbance is frequent. Classically, there is early morning waking, the depressive waking at 4 or 5 in the morning, and being unable to return to sleep. Difficulty in getting off to sleep on going to bed, nightmares and repeated waking from midnight onwards are other sleep patterns in depression.

Bursting into tears during a consultation is a characteristic feature in depression. The flood of tears is short, sharp and unexpected. The episode of crying is usually over in a few minutes and does not prolong the consultation. The woman walks out at the end of the consultation looking into the mirror to adjust her make-up and dry her eyes and states how much better she feels for the happening.

Diurnal mood swing is common. The depressive feels worse in the morning, improving as the day goes on. They often state that 'it is like Monday morning every morning'.

Depression leads to changes in personal social habits and activities. With lack of interest and an inability to concentrate, work efficiency and effectiveness suffer, hobbies are neglected, conversation dries up, television viewing ceases and the victim takes herself off to bed early to suffer alone.

Agitation, irritability, anxieties and fears may all be part of the syndrome. Lack of insight accompanies these symptoms. This lack of insight affects family and friends as well as the victim and the commands 'to pull yourself together' are heard often. These merely add to the anxiety and distress suffered.

A general 'fed-up-ness' with life and a death wish may lead to suicidal talk, gestures and even acts. Suicide is often unpredictable and unexpected in depressives who have been treated and supported for a long time.

Somatic symptoms may be associated or may be the presenting features. Constipation, impotence or frigidity, loss of weight in those who lose interest in eating and a gain in weight in those agitated-depressives in whom compulsive eating is a feature, vague chest pains, dyspepsia and flatulence and pressure headaches may all occur in depressed persons as part of their clinical presentations.

An important clinical sign is the feeling of depression, frustration or agitation that these patients produce in their physicians.

What happens?

Depression is a condition of adult life, but it can occur in children and is often missed.

The onset is at any time during adult life but the peak period for onset is between 30 and 50, particularly in women (Figure 35.2).

Some cases begin in later life, often associated with bereavement.

The annual prevalence rates show peaks between 30 and 60 years but with an appreciable prevalence in the elderly. At all ages

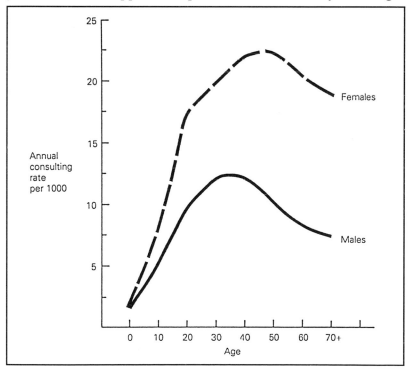

Fig. 35.2—Depression – annual prevalence rates

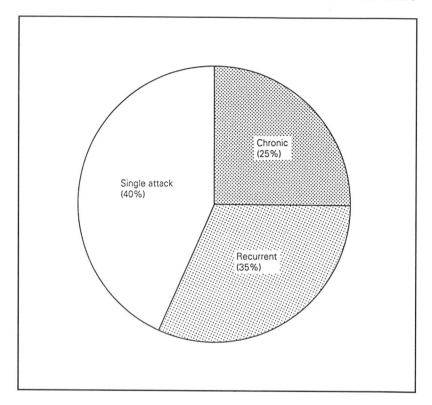

Fig. 35.3—Depression – outcome

the condition is more frequent in females (Figure 35.2).

The course and outcome (Figure 35.3) in depression are unpredictable in the individual case. Each case has to be assessed and considered separately, but the general pattern is as follows.

Of all persons with depression seen in family practice about one-quarter will become chronic cases suffering from persistent or frequent bouts of depression that cause considerable disorganization of personal and family life.

Recurrent bouts of depression at infrequent intervals, longer than 1 year, will occur in one-third. These attacks, whilst disabling and disrupting when they occur, will be limited and between attacks the person will be normal.

A single attack of notable depression will be the pattern in the remaining 40%. The bout of depression is often quite severe and may be prolonged, but once recovered, major attacks do not occur and minor attacks if they do occur tend to be self-limiting and self-managed.

What to do?

Assessment – Is it a depression?

Bearing in mind the wide range of clinical symptoms, it is as well to consider a positive diagnosis of depression when the presentation is somatic rather than emotional.

It is realized that there are no definite objective signs of depression but with the increasing awareness of the possibility of depression as the cause of vague symptoms and with the availability of more specific antidepressant drugs, it is justifiable to carry out a clinical trial of an antidepressant in order to establish the possible diagnosis of depression and to help the patient.

The use of special questionnaires and inventories, whilst valuable for research and for standardization, has little practical application in normal practice.

What type?

Some go to great lengths to separate depression into endogenous and reactive varieties, assuming for them different causations, pathologies, symptoms, course and treatment. It is impossible to be precise and accurate in practice in distinguishing between the two groups. At present when we know so little of the pathogenesis and pathology of the depression, it is best not to try to separate depression into the two varieties but to treat patients as individuals rather than as suffering from reactive or endogenous depression.

Is there a risk of suicide?

The greatest danger in depression is suicide. It would be good if potential suicides could be preselected and protected against themselves. However, there are no reliable criteria on which to base such a preselection.

Accepting that potential suicides cannot be preselected, there have been moves to set up centres for emergency help for possible suicides in an attempt to offer assistance to those contemplating suicide or those depressed. It is assumed that the potential suicide will be prepared to take the step to contact such units by phone or in person, and that he or she knows of their existence, phone number and services.

What help for the family?

Whenever possible a responsible member of the family should be seen for discussion on the nature of the illness and the help and support necessary.

Through such family contacts the personal and other social problems can be discovered, discussed and possibly remedied.

What management?

Depression is often a chronic and recurrent condition. The patient becomes well-known over years. The response to various drugs and other forms of care requires regular evaluation in order to discover what measures are most helpful to the individual patient.

First steps in management of depression are:

(1) Make an early positive diagnosis rather than one of exclusion after lengthy investigations and trials and tribulations of various therapies for possible somatic conditions.

(2) Accept at once that the patient with depression will require regular attention, treatment and support over long periods. It is easier for the physician to accept the diagnosis of depression and to endeavour to treat energetically than to resist or fight the diagnosis and endeavour to treat some pseudo-somatic condition.

(3) Accept with humility and realism that no 'cure' is possible and that one should not resent the need for regular contact and support of individuals who are vulnerable and in need of some help with their life and problems.

(4) The diagnosis having been made it is important to inform the patient that she (or he) is suffering from a 'real' illness for which successful treatment is possible.

It is useful and helpful to go through the chief symptoms of depression to show that the physician knows and understands what the patient is experiencing.

Antidepressant drugs

Most patients with depression will recover naturally without serious difficulties and it is well to remember this before deciding to treat all patients with depression with antidepressants.

If the depression is not severe and if there are underlying causes that can be defined, discussed and corrected, then it is reasonable to wait for a little while (2–3 weeks) in order to see whether there is improvement with support and regular psychotherapy.

Indications for the early use of antidepressants are a history of previous attacks of depression that have responded well to antidepressants; depression that has been present for some weeks and is not improving; and severe symptoms causing much distress.

There are now many antidepressant drugs available and the physician must select two or three and learn how to use them, rather than try out the latest advertized brands.

My first choice is for imipramine or amitriptyline (J.F.). Dosages of these drugs should be increased gradually. Full response may be delayed for 2–3 weeks and once improvement has occurred it is wise to continue for some months before reducing dosage and stopping the drug.

In long-term depressives who respond to tricyclic drugs, it may be necessary to continue with a maintenance dose for a long time in order to prevent recurrences.

Sleep difficulties may require a hypnotic for a short while.

Other measures

In chronic depression electroconvulsive therapy (ECT) still has a real and valuable place and also in some acute and severely depressed patients.

Referral to a psychiatrist is necessary in less than 10% of cases, but it may be required as a therapeutic measure in itself for reassurance and as an alternative source of support in order to arrange ECT or to arrange admission to hospital.

Admission to hospital is necessary in those in whom there is a risk of suicide and where the social and home conditions are difficult.

It is sometimes helpful to refer patients for supportive (GP as well as patient) care when they are not improving and before they enter the category of becoming a 'heart sinker' for the GP.

Practical points

- Important to be alert to the possibility of depression.
- Each GP should develop his or her own plan of management.
- Depression is very prevalent in the community and only 1 in 4 will consult their GP.
- Course appears to be that 40% will suffer a single episode, one-third suffer recurrent episodes and one-quarter will be chronic.
- Assessment is important.
- Most important in management is sympathetic, understanding and regular support; antidepressants are not always necessary; be prepared to refer to psychiatrist before patient becomes a 'heartsinker'; ECT may be effective in severe cases.

SECTION VIII

CNS

CHAPTER 36

DISEASES OF CENTRAL NERVOUS SYSTEM AND SENSE ORGANS

The reason why these conditions are together is because they are classified so in the International Classification of Diseases.

Major neurological diseases, so popular in hospital demonstrations, are uncommon in general practice although the few patients who do suffer do so for a long time (Table 36.1).

However, the less specific and less dramatic disorders of the CNS are more frequent as symptom complexes with few abnormal signs.

Eye and ear problems are relatively common and here also the less serious conditions predominate (Tables 36.2 and 36.3). (See also Chapter 5 for otitis media.)

Patient consulting rates

Table 36.1 shows the likely numbers of consultancy in a year for CNS conditions.

Note the high prevalence of headaches and dizziness. Both of these clinical groups are troublesome to patients, difficult to manage but benign and self-limiting.

TABLE 36.1   Annual consultation rates for CNS disorders

	Persons consulting annually	
Disease	per 2000	per 10 000
Cerebrovascular		
Strokes	12	60
(acute)	(6)	(30)
TIA	4	20
Total	16	80
Migraine	16	80
Headache	34	170
Total	50	250
Dizziness, vertigo	30	150
Epilepsy	12	60
Syncope (faint)	8	40
Total	20	100
Parkinsonism	4	20
Multiple sclerosis	2	10
Brain tumours	1 in 10 yrs	1 in 2 yrs
Motor neurone disease	1 in 20 yrs	1 in 4 yrs
Meningitis	1 in 5 yrs	1

TABLE 36.2   Annual consultation rates for eye diseases

	Persons consulting annually	
Disease	per 2000	per 10 000
Conjunctivitis	56	280
Blepharitis	8	40
Stye	8	40
Total	72	360
Iritis – keratitis	3	15
Cataract	4	20
Glaucoma	2	10
Squint	2	10
Failing vision	10	50
Other	12	60

TABLE 36.3 Annual consultation rates for ear diseases

Disease	Persons consulting annually	
	per 2000	per 10 000
Acute otitis media	92	460
Chronic otitis media	1	5
Otitis externa	22	110
Otosclerosis	1 in 5 yrs	1
Deafness	12	60
Wax	46	230
Others	14	70

Note also the appreciable prevalence of the more chronic disorders such as epilepsy, parkinsonism and multiple sclerosis. Effective management requires planned long-term care by the practice team.

On the other hand, brain tumours at 1 every 10 years, meningitis 1 every 5 years and motor neurone disease 1 every 20 years per GP are rarities.

Sickness/invalidity benefits

The mixture of minor conditions such as headaches and major disorders, strokes and multiple sclerosis, etc., accounts for almost 10% of all days of certified sickness.

Most of the serious disabilities, of course, affect persons beyond retirement age.

Hospital data

7% of all admissions are for these disorders, with strokes and head injuries the largest groups, followed by eye and ear diseases.

Deaths

Strokes are a major cause of death (12% of all deaths) or 2–3 deaths per GP a year.

CHAPTER 37

MIGRAINE

What is it?

'Migraine' is a clinically subjective diagnosis of a quasi-specific type of headache. It is an umbrella term for a symptom spectrum.

Migraine is a complex interplay of neural, vascular and metabolic factors involving neurotransmitters acting on susceptible individuals. 75% of migraine sufferers have a positive family history of migraine (60% maternal and 15% paternal). *Headache* is experienced by four-fifths of the population at sometime and it is likely up to one-fifth of these have migraine.

The *diagnosis* of migraine is based on analysis of symptoms and classified into:

* those without aura (80%)
* those with aura (20%).

Characteristic diagnostic symptoms are:

* headache – unilateral and throbbing
* nausea and/or vomiting
* photophobia and/or phonophobia
* general misery
* prodromal symptoms may be noted.

Triggers include (see also page 352):

- diet – certain foods or missed meals
- excess alcohol – particularly some wines
- lifestyle features
- contraceptive pill or other medication.

Pathophysiology

The traditional view has been that initial vasospasm of the cerebral vessels occurs leading to cerebral ischaemia which accounts for the visual and other types of aura, followed by vasodilatation, which is responsible for the subsequent throbbing headache.

The current view, however, is that the initial change is activation of neurones by a variety of factors, which then results in release of vasoactive substances, such as noradrenaline and serotonin, and it is these substances which subsequently cause the cerebrovascular changes associated with the attack of migraine.

New insights have recently been obtained in relation to the vaso-active neurotransmitters in the aetiology of migraine. One of the most important neurotransmitters is 5-hydroxytryptamine (serotonin), and evidence of a deficiency of 5-HT has been found in migraine. This raises the possibility of the use of 5-HT agonists in the treatment of migraine.

Who gets it and when?

'Migraine' is a common condition but its prevalence depends very much on the diagnostic habits of the clinician making the diagnosis.

Women sufferers outnumber men by over 3:1. *Onset* can be at any age but most often in early adult life and middle age (Figure 37.1). Onset is rare after 60, when an alternative diagnosis should be considered.

Although around 15% of the population suffer from migraine only a minority consult a doctor – most manage their headaches themselves by self-care.

The annual prevalence (Table 37.1) confirms this, less than one person consulting in a week for migraine.

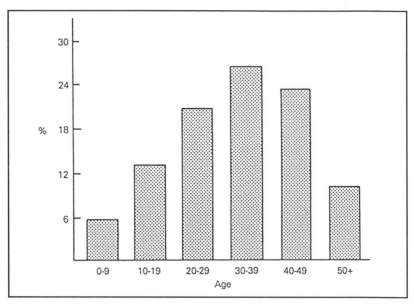

Fig. 37.1—Migraine – age at first diagnosis

TABLE 37.1   Migraine: annual consultation rates

Migraine	per 2000	per 10 000
Annual incidence (new diagnosis)	5	25
Persons consulting annually (prevalence)	40	200
Total suffering from migraine	200	1000
Annual referral to consultant	1	5

The *age-sex prevalence* (Figure 37.2) shows that women consult more than men and that most do so between the ages of 15 and 50.

How does it present?

Types of migraine

- *Classical migraine*: prodromal aura – often visual; headache with nausea/vomiting.
- *Common migraine*: headache without aura.
- *Complicated migraine*: associated with neurological manifestations –

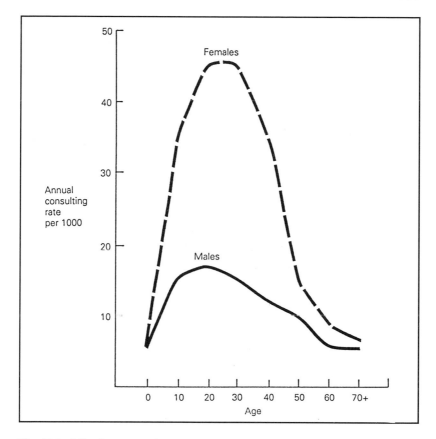

Fig. 37.2—Migraine – annual prevalence

    hemiplegia or hemiparesis
    ophthalmoplegia
    basilar symptoms like diplopia, dysarthria, paraparesis.
- *Migraine equivalents*: prodromata without headache or vomiting – this tends to occur in some chronic migraine sufferers as they grow older – they lose their headache but retain the prodromata.
- *Abdominal migraine*: this diagnosis is often made in children with recurrent abdominal pain and vomiting for which no other cause can be found – the scientific basis for this diagnosis remains dubious.
- *Migrainous neuralgia*: (cluster headache) – the relationship of this condition to the more typical types of migraine remains controversial, since the clinical features have very little in common.

Clinical features

The following clinical features relate to various aspects of migraine.

Periodicity

Migraine occurs in attacks, which are episodic but may occur in clusters. It is unusual for the headache to last longer than a day, but there are some migraine victims in whom a vague background headache persists for many days.

The periodicity is such that it may occur on certain days of the week or month and following certain events. The weekend is a most likely time for a migraine attack.

Triggers

Certain 'trigger' situations are described by migraine victims, particularly if they are asked to record all events on the day of the attack and on the preceding day.

Migraine attacks affect women particularly during their reproductive period and many attacks are related to the menstrual cycle occurring in the premenstrual phase or on the first or second day of menses. Many women find that their migraine attacks are part of the premenstrual tension syndrome, with bloating, increase in weight, pains in the breasts, excessive nervous irritability, tension and depression.

Certain foods may be discovered as triggers and in particular certain chocolates, cheeses, alcoholic drinks, citrus fruits, onions or fried food in general.

A missed meal and a 'lie-in' and later than normal rising may bring on a migraine attack, possibly through effects of hypoglycaemia.

A long and stressful journey, a troublesome meeting at business or with family, a noisy party in a hot and crowded room, an angry altercation or other emotional stresses may all trigger off attacks a day or so later.

Some women find a marked increase in their migraine attacks within a short time of starting to take oral hormone contraceptive tablets.

Combinations of two or more factors may result in attacks where the triggers are difficult to sort out.

Premonitory symptoms

Some migraine sufferers who suffer occasional and infrequent attacks remark how extra well they feel the day before the attack, almost euphoric, only to be let down and struck down on the following day.

Visual symptoms are a warning that were noted by some (one-third) of migraine subjects. Symptoms varied. Floating spots, zig-zags and flashes were those most often described. However, not infrequently a patient appears in great anxiety with a story of partial blindness in one eye followed by a headache.

Parasthesiae and heaviness of one arm and/or the face on the same side may precede the headache. Only rarely are there any motor abnormalities such as transient weakness or paralysis. Such motor symptoms should however raise the probability of a more sinister cause of the symptoms such as an intracranial vascular lesion or tumour.

More observant persons, males and females, may remark on the polyuria that may precede an attack and persist for a few hours. In some this is one of the most dramatic features associated with the headache.

The attack

The headache and malaise are usually there on awakening. The headache is dull, aching, throbbing or sickening and is situated across the front of the head. 'Hemicrania' is not a good description since it is rarely possible for the victim to localize the headache to one side.

The severity of the attack is variable. At one extreme is the person completely incapacitated by a severe headache, vomiting and general physical and emotional collapse, able to lie only in a darkened room, immobile and miserable.

Some attacks are not severe but unpleasant enough to interfere with normal activities.

Accompanying the headache may be feelings of collapse and impending doom and depression. Dizziness or actual vertigo may be present when the victim tries to walk. Light and in particular sunlight may tend to make all the symptoms worse. Nausea and vomiting often occur. Abdominal pains may be a feature of an attack and in young children may replace the headache as the prominent feature.

The 'little belly-achers', children with recurring and periodic abdominal pains, may be a variant of migraine. Certainly these children tend to have a positive family history of migraine and tend to change to headaches following a symptom-free period from 8 to 12 years of age.

Recurrent premonitory symptoms may occur without any subsequent headaches; before labelling these as 'migraine equivalents' intracranial aneurysms or angiomas should be excluded.

Periodic migrainous neuralgia

Periodic migrainous neuralgia is a less common condition, with a prevalence rate of 1 per 1000. It is considered as a migraine equivalent because the symptoms tend to respond specifically to ergot preparations.

It is more common in men than in women.

Its onset is between 30 and 60 years of age and has a characteristic clinical history and course.

The condition occurs in attacks that often come in bouts or clusters. Symptoms consist of sudden, severe, sharp and shooting stabs in the face affecting the nose and eye on the same side.

The attacks tend to occur at the same time often awakening the victim in the early hours of the morning. There is pain on one side of the face often localized discreetly to a small area around the nose and eye. The stabbing pain is accompanied by redness of the eye on the side of the face affected and by watering of the nose.

Each attack lasts about ½–2 hours and then ceases. Attacks tend to occur in bouts or clusters for a week or more, stop, and then recur again after a while until finally ceasing altogether.

Attacks may be prevented by ergot preparations, hence the relationship with migraine.

Migrainous syncope or epilepsy

Two rare variants are *migrainous syncope* or *epilepsy* where there is loss of consciousness during an attack and where the EEG is abnormal – but the EEG is abnormal in one-quarter of all migrainous subjects without loss of consciousness during attacks.

Basilar migraine

Where there is appreciable vertigo, tinnitus and tingling in arms and legs in the premonitory phase it has been suggested that the lesion is sited in the area of the basilar artery and the syndrome has been referred to as *basilar migraine*.

Course

The *course*, once attacks have occurred, is unpredictable at first. Attacks may be infrequent, once a year or less, or they may occur more than once a week. The course, the frequency and severity of attacks and the final outcome follow an individual pattern. But it can be predicted that ultimately, after some years, attacks tend to cease.

What happens?

Migraine does not last for ever. The likely course is for a *period of activity* during which attacks of varying frequency and severity occur for 15–20 years followed by *remission and cessation* (Figure 37.2). This appears to be a natural process related to pathophysiological changes. As noted, 'migraine' is rare in the elderly.

There is a broad *range* of *severity* during the period of activity and only a minority suffer severe and frequent attacks (Figure 37.3).

- *severe* frequent attacks (disruption of life-style)   10%
- *moderate* (at least monthly with inconvenience)   30%
- *minor* (less than once a month and easily controlled)   60%

Follow-up: *20 years from onset* it is likely that persons will have –

- no attacks   65%
- occasional (1–2 per year)   30%
- frequent (more than every 3 months)   5%

What to do?

Assessment

Is it migraine?

Providing that care, attention and time is given to obtaining a history of the attacks, associated features and family and personal circumstances, the diagnosis of migraine should not be difficult.

The only conditions at all likely to cause problems in diagnosis are intracranial vascular lesions such as aneurysms or tumours which by small bleeds can produce symptoms similar to migraine. In these serious conditions there are generally some motor disturbances as well as sensory symptoms.

Why migraine?

Whilst there is no specific cure for migraine, much can be done in preventing attacks by avoiding certain trigger situations and much can be done by instituting treatment early.

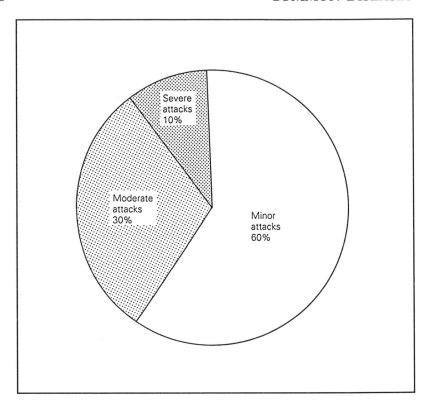

Fig. 37.3—Migraine – severity

In order that the pattern of attacks and possible causal trigger factors may be discovered, the patient and family should undertake recording of each attack in a diary or on specially designed sheets in order to establish the periodicity and true relationships to events such as the menstrual cycle, work, social and leisure habits.

Prepared record cards should be completed for each attack where the victim can go through the events of the preceding day noting any possible causal factors in her habits, diet or general situations, and on the record sheet should be entered, as reminders, trigger factors such as foods, events and situations that can be considered in completing the card.

Simple inspection and analysis of such records will enable definition of possible trigger factors that can be avoided, if discovered.

The aims of sound management are to help the patient to learn how she, or he, might best manage the attacks through prevention or early treatment.

The first basis of good care, then, is to establish a sound doctor–patient relationship whereby the physician's interest is obvious and whence education and guidance can be carried out.

The patient should be told of the nature and likely course of the condition and of the principles of management.

Detection of trigger factors

As noted (on pages 349–352) certain trigger factors can be defined and once defined, steps can be taken to avoid them in an attempt to prevent attacks. Some success will always be achieved but even when triggers are defined and avoided attacks can and will occur.

Management of migraine

General measures

- Patient education on the nature of the condition and the likely course, also on the benefits and the limitations of treatment.
- Identification and avoidance if possible of any trigger factors, e.g. stress, food, alcohol, chocolate, etc.
  In cases of premenstrual migraine, a diuretic taken in the premenstrual week may prevent attacks.
- Avoid any drugs which may precipitate migraine, e.g. contraceptives, vasodilators.

Treatment of an attack

Mild attack

- Simple analgesic first, e.g. aspirin 600–900 mg or paracetamol 1 gram.
- Drug absorption from the stomach is slowed in an attack of migraine; the measures which can improve gastric absorption of analgesics are:
  use of a soluble preparation of the analgesic
  metoclopramide 10 mg (Maxolon) or domperidone 10–20 mg (Motilium) given with the analgesic. An additional advantage of metoclopramide or domperidone when used in migraine is their anti-emetic action.

Severe attack

- Rest in a darkened room.
- Use of an *ergot* preparation:
  oral   Cafergot 1–4 tablets/day
  suppository   Cafergot 1–2 suppositories

aerosol   Medihaler ergotamine 1–6 puffs/day
sublingual   Lingraine 2–6 mg/day
side-effects   nausea/vomiting
                 abdominal and muscular cramps
                 aggravation of headache sometimes
                 gangrene with overdose – more than
                     8 mg/day or 12 mg/week

- *Sumatriptan* – this is a new 5-hydroxytryptamine agonist which has been found to be very effective in relieving headache, vomiting and photophobia in severe attacks of migraine. Its use is based on recent research which shows depletion of 5-HT levels in migraine. In clinical trials the response rate with subcutaneous injection of sumatriptan has been 70%. Oral trials are continuing. One possible hazard recently highlighted in the British Medical Journal[1,2] has been the occurrence of coronary vasospasm with ECG changes of ischaemia after subcutaneous injection of sumatriptan, which may inhibit its use in some patients.

Prophylactic drugs in migraine

Prophylaxis is desirable if attacks are occurring more than once a week.

Four types of drug are currently available for prophylactic treatment:

Beta-blockers

About 70% of patients benefit from propranolol (Inderal) 10–20 mg t.d.s.

Serotonin antagonists

Pizotifen (Sanomigran) 2–6 mg/24 h is first choice. Up to 80% of patients have long-lasting relief. It can be used in classic or common migraine, and also in cluster headache. Possible side-effects include stimulation of appetite with resultant gain in weight, drowsiness and problems with glaucoma and urinary retention because of its anticholinergic effect.

Methysergide (Deseril) may be tried in very resistant patients – it is effective in up to 65% of patients. The main problem with methysergide is its high incidence of side-effects, in up to 40% of patients; these include nausea, insomnia and – potentially most hazardous – retroperitoneal fibrosis with ureteric obstruction, fibrosis of the pleura and even occasional involvement of heart valves. If used, it should be used for limited periods only and under hospital supervision.

Clonidine (Dixarit) is of limited value in migraine because of minimal prophylactic effect and the occurrence of depression and insomnia with this drug.

Calcium-channel blockers

There is some evidence that verapamil and nifedipine may be useful in migraine prophylaxis.

Tricyclic antidepressants

May be of value in some patients. Amitriptyline 10 mg at night increasing if necessary up to 75 mg at night.

Practical points

- Migraine is a symptom complex in the spectrum of headaches.
- It is said to affect 5–10% of the population at some time but the annual patient consulting rates are much less because most victims manage their headaches themselves. A practice with 2000 patients can expect 5 new cases and 40 persons consulting annually.
- The clinical features are unilateral headache, nausea and vomiting and in some a preceding aura.
- Most migraneurs start attacks in their teens or early adult life. There is a strong family history and women are more affected than men (3 : 1).
- After a period of 15–20 years, attacks tend to cease naturally.
- In management general advice on avoidance of attacks and explanation of likely prognosis and outcome are important.
- Specific treatment has to be tailored to the individual patient and severity of attacks. Most are mild–moderate and can be controlled with analgesics. For more severe attacks ergot preparations have been traditional but now there is sumatriptan.
- Prophylaxis for severe attacks includes use of beta-blockers and pizotifen.

References

1. Willett F, Curzon N, Adams J, *et al.*, Coronary vasospasm induced by subcutaneous sumatriptan. *Br. Med. J. 1992*; 304: 1415.
2. Stricher BHC. Coronary vasospasm and sumatriptan. *Br. Med. J. 1992*; 305: 118.

CHAPTER 38

EPILEPSY AND CONVULSIONS

What is it?

Epilepsy and convulsions are symptoms of some underlying disorder, though admittedly in two-thirds no cause can be determined.

They are characterized by sudden, and often repeated, fits or seizures – ranging from *minor* 'absences', sensory disturbances, motor jerks or twitches, to major convulsions with loss of consciousness. In some individuals the episodes include psycho-emotional changes.

The *causes* are:

- non-detected   65%
- vascular   15%
- alcohol excess   5%
- cerebral tumour   5%
- post-trauma   2%
- others such as neonatal and
  metabolic causes   8%

The *clinical presentation* also ranges widely:

- febrile convulsions [1 in 20 children]   30%
- true epilepsy   50%
- possible epilepsy   20%

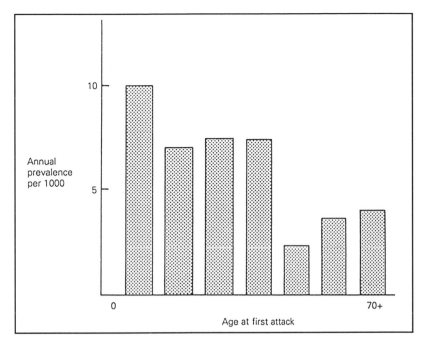

Fig. 38.1—Epilepsy – age at first attack

The *types* of attacks also vary and a person may suffer more than one:

- generalized   50%
- partial/focal   30%
- mixed   20%

Who and when?

Figure 38.1 shows that epilepsy can *commence* at any age but most often in childhood. Males and females are equally affected.

Figure 38.2 shows that *prevalence* of *attacks* also is most likely in childhood and young adults.

The *prevalence in practice* (Table 38.1) shows that numbers are significant and of course management is long-term and may be difficult.

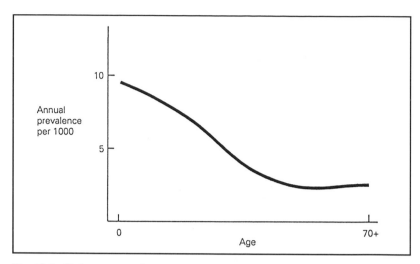

Fig. 38.2—Epilepsy – prevalence

TABLE 38.1   Epilepsy: prevalence in general practice

Epilepsy and convulsions	per 2000	per 10 000
Annual incidence (new diagnoses)	1–2	5–8
Annual prevalence (persons consulting)	10–15	50–75
All persons with past / present history (active and inactive)	50–60	250–300

Note: 1 in 20 children have a febrile convulsion.

How do they present?

Faint or fit?

To differentiate epilepsy from other causes of loss of consciousness, the factors which need to be assessed are:

- events preceding the loss of consciousness (aura);
- period of unconsciousness;
- period after recovery of consciousness.

Preceding events

- Unilateral neurological symptoms suggests epilepsy and indicates the likely site of origin in the brain.

- Auditory, olfactory or taste hallucinations suggest temporal lobe epilepsy.
- A syncopal attack is suggested by:
light-headedness
pallor
nausea
sweating
palpitations

During period of unconsciousness

- Grand mal epilepsy – tonic/clonic phase few minutes only.
- Epileptic 'absences' – few seconds only.
- Associated features in epilepsy
tongue biting
incontinence of urine
likelihood of injury.
- Convulsions may occasionally occur in a syncopal attack but are briefer than epilepsy, less violent and there is less chance of injury.

After recovery of consciousness

- Headache, drowsiness and confusion are very suggestive of epilepsy.
- There are very few after-effects following a syncopal attack.
- 'Automatic' behaviour may occur following an epileptic attack but is very rare: the behaviour may be bizarre or purposeful.
- Rarely, temporary paralysis may occur following an epileptic attack (Todd's paralysis) – this takes the form of a focal neurological deficit lasting up to 24 hours.

Other factors

Other clues which may be helpful in differentiating epilepsy from syncope are:

- family history of epilepsy
- past history of birth injury or head injury
- past history of complicated febrile convulsions
- a past history of hypertension, coronary, cerebrovascular or peripheral arterial disease suggests the possibility of a syncopal attack
- attacks occurring at night or when the patient is recumbent are more likely to be epileptic.

Clinical types

The following are some features of the various types but there may be a mixture in individuals.

Generalized

- Grand mal: aura followed by cry, loss of consciousness, tonic–clonic spasms and after-effects including headache, confusion, drowsiness and, rarely, automatism.
- Absence (perit mal): transient and brief (5–10 seconds) with some alteration in consciousness, such as sudden blankness or staring and cessation of activity.
- Myoclonic jerks: sudden brief episodes of generalized muscle twitching but no alteration of consciousness – 'salaam' may occur from flexion of trunk.
- Akinetic epilepsy: sudden transient loss of muscle tone leading to a fall (a type of 'drop attack').

Partial–focal

Presentation depends on site of epilepogenic focus.

- Partial motor (Jacksonian): often in the hand with twitching of thumb and index finger spreading up arm to face. This may be followed by loss of consciousness and convulsion. May also be followed by transient monoparesis (Todd's paralysis).
- Partial sensory: similar spread to Jacksonian but only parasthesiae.
- Partial autonomic: epigastric sensation, pallor or flushing and hair standing up.
- Psychomotor (partial/mixed): *déjà vu*, unusual smells, emotional, lip smacking, hallucinations, aimless or automatic behaviour (may be used as defence in criminal activity).

Febrile convulsions

- Peak at 9 months – 2 years.
- Triggered by fever in susceptible children, often with a family history.
- Jerking followed by generalized convulsions and loss of consciousness.
- Most attacks last only a few minutes.
- If prolonged then may be due to some intracerebral condition such as meningitis or encephalitis.

What happens?

Because of the various types and causes the course and outcome vary.

Children

- Neonatal convulsions with brain damage – the prognosis is bad.
- Febrile convulsions – 95% will cease after the age of 3 or so and only 5% continue epileptic attacks.

Adults

The outlook is much better than is generally assumed and only a minority continue attacks and require long-term medication.

After 10 years from first attack:

- 1 in 2 will have no attacks
- 1 in 3 will have 1 or 2 per year
- 1 in 6 will have more than 2 per year
- 1 in 20 will be seriously disturbed.

It is believed that early effective treatment with appropriate drugs will prevent recurrences.

Without treatment of first attacks:

- 60% will recur in first year
- 80% will recur in 3 years.

What to do?

Assessment

Is it epilepsy?

A label of epilepsy is a serious matter and the diagnosis should not be made unless there is good evidence for the diagnosis, supported by an abnormal electro-encephalogram.

Suggestive clinical features of a diagnosis of epilepsy are – a positive family history, nocturnal attacks, convulsive movements, tongue biting and incontinence during an attack and odd behaviour after an attack.

What possible causes?

Although in most epileptic convulsive disorders there are no major underlying causes, a search has to be made. In general, serious causes are more likely in the neonatal period and in those whose attacks begin after the age of 40.

Of the serious causes that account for 5% of all epileptics the following are most likely – post-traumatic, neonatal and later brain injuries; intracranial tumours; cerebral atherosclerosis; meningitis; and various metabolic disorders such as diabetes, uraemia and alcoholism. Idiopathic epilepsy may be triggered off by situations such as fasting and missing meals, premenstrual tension and fluid retention, visual flicker, excessive alcohol, lack of sleep and fever.

Management

It is easier to control epileptic attacks than to help and manage the social problems that sometimes face the epileptic.

Epilepsy still is an unacceptable condition for many employers. The dangers are clear for an epileptic engaging in potentially risky occupations such as driving, engineering or any job where sudden loss of consciousness will create danger for the epileptic and others and no epileptic should engage in such work. But many employers are reluctant to accept epileptics in sedentary office, agricultural or other work that is safe to all, because they are fearful of attacks disrupting their organization and fearful of a disease to which much mysticism is still attached.

Epilepsy therefore is a serious handicap and the diagnostic label must not be attached too readily.

Children with febrile convulsions usually do not suffer epilepsy in later life. Less than 5% of children with febrile convulsions suffer convulsions as adults. It is quite wrong to label children with febrile convulsions as epileptics.

Likewise most children with petit mal attacks will not suffer major epileptic attacks as adults and it is wrong to call these 'epileptics'.

The natural history of epilepsy, in J.F.'s practice, was of a condition that was easy to control and that one-half cease to suffer attacks spontaneously. Only 15% of all adult epileptics suffered more than 2 attacks per year and only 5% of all epileptics required special care because of serious mental and physical disabilities (Figure 38.3).

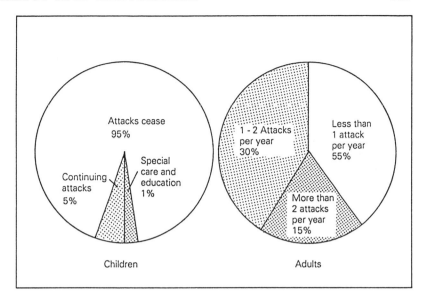

Fig. 38.3—Outcomes of epilepsy

Social problems

In addition to problems of occupation, epileptics are often faced with personal problems such as marriage, life insurance policies and driving licences.

Unless there is a family history of epilepsy in both prospective husband and wife, then there is no good reason for advising against marriage and childbearing.

If epileptic attacks are well controlled over some years then it should be possible to obtain good life insurance cover and driving licences.

Investigation of epilepsy

(1) *Physical examination* is usually unhelpful in the diagnosis of epilepsy, but occasionally there are some clues that can be found (Figure 38.4).

(2) *Electro-encephalogram (EEG)* – it is important to note that a normal EEG does not exclude epilepsy. In the great majority of diagnoses of epilepsy, the diagnosis is made on a careful clinical history alone.

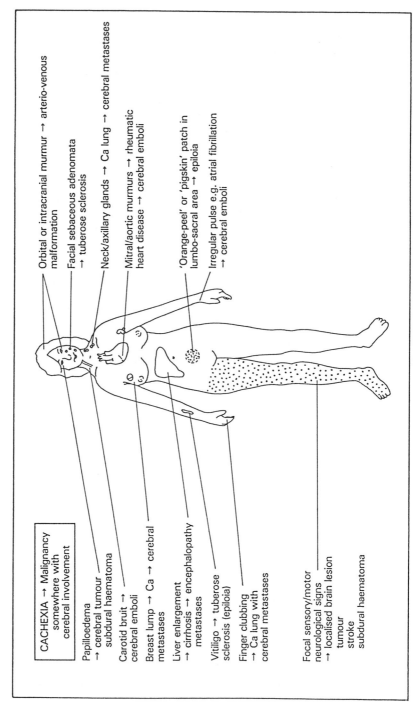

Fig. 38.4—Possible clinical findings in a person with epilepsy

Orbital or intracranial murmur → arterio-venous malformation

Facial sebaceous adenomata → tuberose sclerosis

Neck/axillary glands → Ca lung → cerebral metastases

Mitral/aortic murmurs → rheumatic heart disease → cerebral emboli

'Orange-peel' or 'pigskin' patch in lumbo-sacral area → epiloia

Irregular pulse e.g. atrial fibrillation → cerebral emboli

CACHEXIA → Malignancy somewhere with cerebral involvement

Papilloedema → cerebral tumour subdural haematoma

Carotid bruit → cerebral emboli

Breast lump → Ca → cerebral metastases

Liver enlargement → cirrhosis → encephalopathy metastases

Vitiligo → tuberose sclerosis (epiloia)

Finger clubbing → Ca lung with cerebral metastases

Focal sensory/motor neurological signs → localised brain lesion tumour stroke subdural haematoma

Functions of the EEG:
  adds weight to clinical diagnosis
  helps to classify the type of epilepsy
  may show changes of an underlying organic lesion, e.g.
  brain tumour.
- 10–15% of the population have an abnormal EEG – this is usually a mild abnormality of no clinical significance.
- 1% of the population have more specific changes of spikes or spike-and-waves indicative of epilepsy.
- 50% of epileptic patients have a normal EEG between attacks.

(3) *Ambulatory cardiac monitoring* may be helpful if a syncopal attack due to heart block is suspected.

(4) A *CT brain scan* is necessary if organic disease is suspected to exclude a potentially-operable brain tumour, and also to pick up cerebrovascular lesions. It is also necessary in new onset epilepsy in adult life since 10% of these patients have a brain tumour.

(5) A recently-introduced test of measuring *prolactin levels* in the blood after a suspected epileptic attack can help to differentiate it from a pseudo-seizure, as there is a transient rise of the prolactin level 15–20 minutes after a grand mal or partial complex seizure without loss of consciousness.

NB – routine investigation of skull X-ray, haematology or blood biochemistry are usually of no value in the diagnosis of epilepsy.

Specific drug treatment

Initiation of treatment

There is still some doubt about whether to start drug treatment for epilepsy after one attack. One view suggests that treatment should be started if there is no doubt about the diagnosis of an epileptic fit and the circumstances of the patient's life means that there is danger of a serious injury if another fit occurs. The more general view, however, is that drug treatment should be withheld until it is seen whether another fit is going to occur.

Principles

- Know a few drugs well.
- Use only one drug at a time.
- Increase to maximum tolerable dose before accepting that the drug is ineffective.

- Do not forget to monitor the blood level to see that it is within the therapeutic range.

Grand mal attacks

- First choice:
  phenytoin (Epanutin)
  carbamazepine (Tegretol)
  sodium valproate (Epilim)
- Second choice:
  primidone (Mysoline)
  vigabatrin (Sabril)
  phenobarbitone
  clonazepam (Rivotril)

Petit mal (absences) and myoclonic seizures

- First choice:
  sodium valproate
  ethosuximide (Zarontin)
- Second choice:
  clonazepam

Partial simple and complex seizures

- First choice:
  carbamazepine
  phenytoin
- Second choice:
  sodium valproate
  primidone
  clonazepam
  phenobarbitone
  vigabatrin

Side-effects of drugs

Unfortunately all anticonvulsant drugs have possible side-effects:

- over sedation – phenobarbitone and primidone
- rashes – phenobarbitone and phenytoin
- loss of hair – sodium valproate
- hirsutism – phenytoin
- gum hyperplasia – phenytoin
- ataxia – phenobarbitone, phenytoin, carbamazepine
- macrocytic anaemia – phenobarbitone and phenytoin
- foetal abnormalities (in pregnant women) – phenytoin and sodium valproate.

Failure of treatment to control the attacks

Possible reasons:

- the commonest cause is failure to take the drugs regularly or at all
- psychological problems which influence compliance
- the diagnosis may be wrong and the 'fits' not due to epilepsy at all
- the fits may be caused by a progressive underlying organic lesion, especially a brain tumour.

Withdrawal of successful anticonvulsant therapy

The risk of relapse of the epilepsy in patients successfully treated who have had no attacks for the previous 2 years is from 20% to 50%. The longer the period free of attacks the more likely there is to be permanent suppression of the fits after discontinuing treatment.

The factors which may help in deciding to discontinue treatment include:

- With a long history of epilepsy the fit-free period should be at least 2 years. With a more recent history and successful control, treatment can be withdrawn if required after a year free of attacks.
- With partial seizures, treatment should be continued long-term – withdrawal is undesirable.
- Always consider carefully the possible adverse results of withdrawal in individual patients if a fit were to recur.

Epilepsy in the elderly

- Prevalence of epilepsy in the elderly is 6–8 per 10 000.
- Cerebrovascular disease is the commonest cause – the epilepsy may either follow a stroke, or it may be the first indication of underlying cerebrovascular disease.
- The epilepsy is caused by brain tumours in 10–15%.
- Alcohol and prescribed drugs may also be contributory factors.
- Diagnosis is difficult in the elderly because of:
  poor history
  frequency of heart and cerebral disease.

Practical points

- 'Epilepsy' is a symptom, not a disease.
- In 65% of cases no cause is found. In 15%, mostly in the elderly, the cause is cardiovascular. Cerebral tumour is the cause in only 5% of new fits.
- A GP with 2000 patients may expect 1–2 new cases annually, 10–15 epileptics consulting and another 40–50 persons with a past-history but no problems.
- Diagnosis at onset is not easy.
- Clinical types range widely and classification is unhelpful in practice. Types are generalized, partial, mixed and febrile.
- Outcomes depend on types and causes but are better than generally asumed.
  After 10 years from first fit (in adults)
  1 in 2 have no fits
  1 in 3 have 1–2 fits a year
  1 in 6 have more than 2 fits a year
  1 in 20 are seriously disabled.
- Management includes:
  early accurate diagnosis
  general support and education
  protection regarding occupation, driving and social activities but with as normal a life as possible
  prevention of attacks by drugs.
- Anticonvulsants – there are many to choose from. Get to know a few well and endeavour to use one at a time where possible and to achieve maximal dosage before changing. Note, appreciable side-effects.

CHAPTER 39

STROKES

What are they?

Strokes result from interference with cerebral circulation from a variety of causes leading to global or focal disturbance of cerebral function.

The causes may be atheromatous changes in the cerebral arteries, emboli from the left side of the heart or haemorrhage either into the brain (intracerebral) or around it (subarachnoid) from the weakened walls of cerebral blood vessels from congenital or acquired causes.

In completed strokes the clinical features persist for longer than 24 hours; in transient ischaemic attacks (TIA) they clear within 24 hours.

The proportions of the pathological types (Figure 39.1) are:

- cerebral infarction   65%
- cerebral haemorrhage   20%
- TIA   10%
- others (e.g. tumours)   5%

Who gets them and when?

Strokes, particularly cerebral infarction, are conditions generally associated with ageing; cerebral haemorrhage and TIA tend to

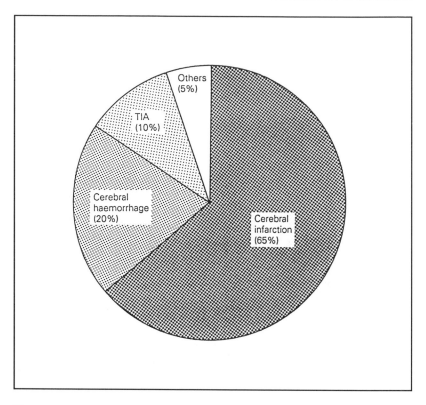

Fig. 39.1—Strokes – proportions of the pathological types

affect younger persons (Table 39.1 and Figure 39.2).

TABLE 39.1   Annual incidence of strokes per 10 000

	Age					
	under 55	55–64	65–74	75–84	85+	All ages
Annual incidence per 10 000	3	25	100	150	250	20

The number of persons who are likely to develop a stroke (incidence), numbers consulting per year (prevalence) and those dying and disabled per 2000 and per 10 000 are in Table 39.2.

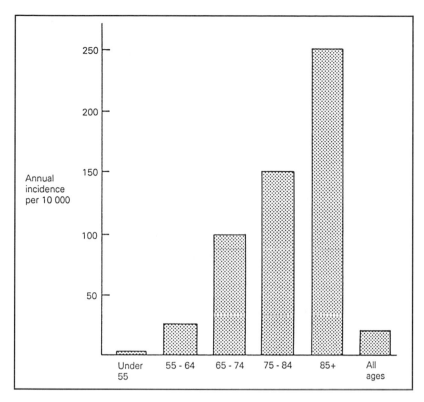

Fig. 39.2—Strokes – annual incidence

TABLE 39.2   Strokes: incidence and prevalence per 2000, and 10 000 persons

	per 2000	per 10 000
Annual incidence (new)	3–4	15–20
Annual persons consulting (prevalence) (old and new cases)	15–20	75–100
Annual deaths	3	15
Disabled from stroke (moderate/severe)	10	50

Whilst numbers of new cases are not great, those of survivors, many of whom are disabled, are appreciable.

Associated with strokes are high blood pressure (× 5 the rate in non-stroke persons) and ischaemic heart disease (× 6 the rate in non-stroke persons).

Risk factors

- Increasing age
- hypertension – at >110 mmHg diastolic pressure incidence is 15 times greater than with a diastolic pressure of 80 mm
- smoking
- lower socio-economic class.

Pathogenesis of stroke

Thromboembolism

Accounts for up to 33% of strokes; most originate in the left ventricle or left atrium and may be associated with:

- diseased valves – including prolapsed mitral valves
- acute myocardial infarction
- left ventricular aneurysm
- atrial fibrillation from whatever cause
- carotid atheroma in the neck.

Cerebral atherosclerosis

Underlying pathology is atherosclerosis, and the stroke is precipitated by platelet aggregation leading to clot formation.

Primary intracranial haemorrhage

Usually the result of hypertension and the development of microaneursyms (Charcot-Bouchard aneurysms).

Usual sites

- basal ganglia
- brain stem
- cerebellum.

Subarachnoid haemorrhage

Usually due to a ruptured berry aneurysm in the circle of Willis, often on the anterior communicating artery.

Less common causes

- Blood abnormalities, e.g. polycythaemia
- Vasculitis, e.g. collagen disease
- Malignancy.

Transient ischaemic attacks

Most are from small emboli which lyse rapidly. The majority of these emboli originate in the carotid arteries in the neck, though any of the causes above in the section on thromboembolism may apply.

How do they present?

Clinical features

The most useful practical approach to assessing presenting clinical features in strokes is that which combines severity with some prognositc guide.

Three grades may be defined:

Severe grade includes those who are unconscious and remain so for more than an hour; those with hemiplegia; and those with persisting major neurological disturbances.

Moderate grades are those in whom the persisting neurological disturbances are less disabling, such as weakness in one limb or visual disturbance in one eye, or in whom major defects begin to improve within the first week.

Minor grades are the transient neurological defects which although producing minor long-term functional disability, are nevertheless of great potential importance as early warnings of more major strokes to come. These minor and transient ischaemic attacks may predate imminent more complete strokes. One in 3 develop stroke within 5 years.

Presentation of cerebral thrombosis/infarction

Middle cerebral artery – commonest artery affected:

- patient often awakens with a stroke
- homonymous hemianopia
- spastic hemiplegia/hemianaesthesia
- dysphasia if right-sided stroke
- occasionally onset with an epileptic fit.

Anterior cerebral artery:

- hcmiplcgia – lcg > arm
- apraxia
- motor dysphasia
- disorder of micturition.

Posterior cerebral artery:

- homonymous hemianopia
- crossed paralysis – cranial nerve paresis on side of the thrombosis and hemiparesis on opposite side
- diplopia, vertigo, ataxia, nystagmus.

Presentation of cerebral haemorrhage

- Most occur in the internal capsule.
- Most lose consciousness.
- Initial epileptic fit common.
- Hemiplegia – flaccid at first and later spastic.
- Often raised intracranial pressure with papilloedema.
- Frequently progressive – 50% die within a few days.

Other sites of haemorrhage:

- *Brain stem*
  hyperpyrexia
  pinpoint pupils
  Cheyne-Stokes respiration
  bilateral involvement of cranial nerves and pyramidal tracts.
- *Cerebellum*
  occipital headache
  vomiting and vertigo
  ataxia
  contralateral hemiplegia.

Complications of stroke

- *Cerebral oedema* – suspect if patient is lucid for 24 hours then progressively loses consciousness.
- *Immobility* leading to:
  pneumonia – especially if swallowing difficulties
  oedema of paralysed limbs
  venous thrombosis
  pressure sores
  shoulder pain on the hemiplegic side.

What happens?

The overall life expectancy of a first stroke patient is poor – over the following 10 years there is a five-fold increased risk of dying, compared with a non-stroke person.

The likely outcome following an acute stroke is:

Deaths

> - 25% will die in first month.
> - Another 15% will die in next 11 months.
> - *Thus 40% will die in first year.*

[Death rates are higher in cerebral haemorrhage than in cerebral infarction]

Survivors

> - 1 in 2 survivors will have minor or no disabilities.
> - 1 in 2 survivors will have considerable disabilities.
> - 1 in 10 survivors will require long-term care in hospital or nursing home.

Hemiplegia is the most likely disability following cerebral infarction.

The likely outcome is:

- 70% will be able to walk
- 15% will recover useful hand/finger function
- when affected, recovery of speech in less than one-half.

Recovery is likely in the first 2 months after acute stroke – but slow after this period.

TIA is associated with a 5-fold extra risk of developing a stroke within the next 10 years and a 3-fold extra risk of death (most from myocardial infarction).

Deaths from strokes have declined considerably in most countries over the past 25 years.

Carers

Since one-half of stroke survivors are left disabled they will need considerable help, care and support at home producing strains on personal and community carers.

What to do?

Assessment

Is the diagnosis of 'stroke' correct?

'Stroke' is a broad term that incorporates the various clinical entities that result from obstruction of cerebral arterial blood flow. Other conditions such as intracranial neoplasms and other space-occupying lesions, metabolic disturbances such as diabetes and porphyria, and infections may produce similar clinical features.

Home or hospital?

The less severely disturbed cases can be managed at home in the initial stages.

Coma and severe disabilities needing skilled nursing will have to be admitted to hospital.

Where diagnosis is in doubt hospitalization will be necessary.

Home care is possible when the patient is not severely handi-capped, when he can get out of bed and walk with assistance, where there are friends and relatives to help in nursing and where home nurses can provide skilled assistance and support; and where the family and patient are keen for home care.

Investigations in stroke

CT or NMR X-rays – haemorrhage can be seen within a few hours but may be normal for the first 24 hours in an ischaemic stroke. If the test is delayed for over 2 weeks, then it may not be possible to distinguish infarction from haemorrhage.

This investigation is the most useful one in stroke, and is essential if any form of anticoagulant treatment is going to be considered.

The other valuable function of the test is to pick up a cerebral tumour or a subarachnoid haemorrhage.

The scan may be normal if there is a small deep infarct or if the lesion is in the posterior fossa.

Blood clotting parameters – this may be useful in intracranial haemorrhage, the most important test being the prothrombin index if a patient is already on warfarin, e.g. for atrial fibrillation. There are other more sophisticated measurements, e.g. proteins C and S, antithrombin III, but these disorders leading to cerebral haem-orrhage are rare.

Carotid angiography – this is associated with a 1% risk of stroke. The indications are:

• if surgery is being considered for a severe carotid artery stenosis in the neck

- for subarachnoid haemorrhage
- progressive and recurrent cerebrovascular symptoms in a younger patient, to see if there is an underlying vascular abnormality which may be the cause.

Lumbar puncture – this is only necessary if:

- subarachnoid haemorrhage is suspected and the CT scan is either not available or it is normal
- if meningitis is suspected.

Management

Principles

- Prevent by controlling raised blood pressure (primary).
- Good nursing in acute phase.
- Prevent and treat complications.
- Rehabilitate.
- Prevent recurrence (secondary).

Special aids and services

In long-term care of permanently disabled patients with strokes a careful early assessment and review should be made, in each case, of the available social and allied services that may be brought in to help the patient at home.

For example, simple aids to daily living in re-adapting the home for the disabled stroke victim include putting in rails for the hemiplegic to hold on to with his non-paralysed hand, altering toilet seats, installing aids to enable the person to bath or to take a shower independently and in obtaining the many gadgets to help in eating, dressing and walking.

Acute phase

The first aim must be to *maintain life* in those who are unconscious or severely affected and these must be admitted to hospital as emergencies.

The next objective is to take steps to *maintain and restore function*. This requires careful attention to paralysed limbs in order to prevent contractures and deformities and to encourage movement power. Initially, the case should be supervised by a physiotherapist or nurse but the aim must be to teach the patient and family to carry out the exercises themselves all through the day.

Communications and relations with the family are important in order to inform and prepare them for the likely course and outcome, and for any adjustments and alterations that may be required for the patient at home. Alternatively, arrangements may have to be considered for a long-stay unit when the disabilities are great and recovery incomplete.

Specific treatment

Admission to hospital is not essential.

Treatment of cerebral oedema has been tried with a variety of agents, such as mannitol, glycerol, steroids, naftidrofuryl, but there is no convincing evidence from properly controlled clinical trials that any of these measures produce any significant benefit.

Anticoagulation is useful if there are frequent TIAs or if there is stepwise progression of the stroke. It is important to ensure that a cerebral haemorrhage is excluded by a CT scan if anticoagulation is considered in stroke.

Aspirin may be of value if given in the early stages of stroke, but more clinical trials are needed to assess this properly.

Nimodipine, a calcium channel blocker, is of value in subarachnoid haemorrhage, but is of no benefit in ischaemic stroke.

Control of hypertension should be done carefully and only if the diastolic pressure is over 120 mm. Lowering of the blood pressure should be slow with an oral agent, otherwise there is risk of increasing ischaemic damage to the brain.

Neurosurgery in stroke

The main indications are:

* subarachnoid haemorrhage;
* the removal of cerebellar haematomata;
* removal of cerebral haematomata in younger patients is currently being researched.

After care

One-half of survivors will be severely disabled and require considerable care and support.

Initially intensive physiotherapy and rehabilitation are necessary at a stroke unit or centre.

Ideally, where possible, the stroke victim should eventually be at home with full support of social aids and services.

Aids may be required to adapt the home, meals-on-wheels may be needed, home-help and home nursing services may be helpful and regular visits by the general practice team to encourage the patient and maintain communication links.

Rehabilitation of the family is as important as that of the stroke victim.

Prevention

Can anything be done to prevent strokes before they happen (primary prevention)?

Probably, the best hope is the control of high blood pressure, in particular in those under 60, and especially in males.

There is no known way of controlling atherosclerosis, as yet. Aneurysms of intracranial arteries cannot be treated before they bleed, but 'little bleeds' may be a warning and if the aneurysm can be diagnosed at this stage definitive treatment may prevent catastrophic subarachnoid haemorrhage.

Cerebral embolism may be prevented by life-long anticoagulation in persons following cardiac surgery, and in those with persistent and uncontrolled cardiac arrhythmias.

Secondary prevention after a stroke

- Stop smoking.
- Control hypertension.
- Control hyperlipidaemia.
- Aspirin:
  clear benefit in TIAs
  probably also prevents recurrence of stroke – dose remains controversial but the consensus seems to be that 300 mg/day is probably best.
- anticoagulation – indicated in:
  valvular heart disease
  atrial fibrillation
  recurrent TIAs
  thrombotic states, e.g. protein C or S deficiency.

Practical points

- Strokes result from interference with cerebral circulation leading to temporary or permanent disturbances of cerebral function.
- Pathological types include cerebral infarction (65%), cerebral haemorrhage (20%), TIA (10%) and others such as tumours and other space-occupying lesions (5%).
- Strokes increase with age, particularly those from cerebral infarction. Cerebral haemorrhage and TIA tend to occur in younger persons.
- A GP with 2000 patients can expect each year 4 new strokes, 3 deaths from strokes (new and old cases) and 10 persons disabled from strokes.
- The prognosis of stroke is not good; one-quarter die in the first month after a stroke and 40% will be dead within a year. Of survivors, one-half will have minor disabilities and the other half will be moderately or severely disabled. One in 10 of survivors will require long-term care in a nursing home or hospital.
- After hemiplegia – 70% will be able to walk, 15% will recover some use of the hands and one-half of those affected will recover speech.
- After TIA, one-third will suffer a stroke unless effective anticoagulation is achieved.
- All but minor cases should be admitted to hospital – to maintain life and achieve early rehabilitation, and in a few instances neurosurgery may be indicated.
- Long-term care at home requires assistance and support of carers as well as the stroke victim.
- Secondary prevention should include non-smoking, control of hypertension, aspirin for anticoagulation and regular physical exercise.

SECTION IX

ENDOCRINOLOGY

CHAPTER 40

ENDOCRINE AND METABOLIC DISORDERS – THE CLINICAL SPECTRUM

Clinically exotic endocrine disorders affecting adrenal and pituitary glands are uncommon but diabetes, thyroid disorders and obesity are very much part of general practice. Since they are long-term conditions, there is need for appropriate planned and shared care within the practice and in collaboration with specialists.

Patient consulting rates

Table 40.1 shows the annual numbers of patients consulting for these conditions. Probably they are an underestimate of the true prevalence in the community. Thus it is likely that at least 10% of adults are moderately *overweight* and 1% considerably over-weight. This means some 200 in a practice of 2000, whereas only 30 consult in a year.

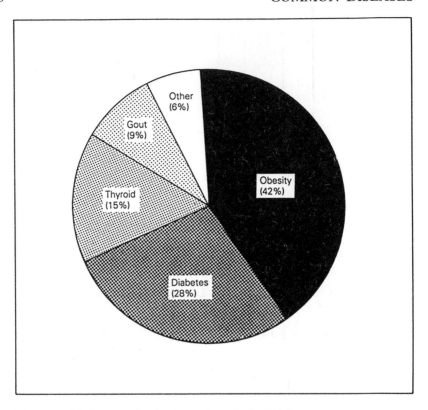

Fig. 40.1—Distribution of endocrine and metabolic disorders

TABLE 40.1   Annual consultation rates for endocrine and metabolic disorders

Disease	Persons consulting annually	
	per 2000	per 10 000
Obesity	30	150
Diabetes	20	100
Thyroid		
hyperthyroid	5	25
hypothyroid	6	30
Total	11	55
Gout	6	30
Other	4	20
Total	71	355

Likewise, it is likely that the prevalence of *diabetes* in the community is almost 2% but only 1% (20 per 2000) consult annually suggesting many undiagnosed, presumably mild or borderline, diabetics.

Thyroid disorders are not uncommon, over 10 consulting in a year, one-half hyperthyroid or goitre and one-half hypothyroid. It is likely, also, that there are some undiagnosed cases in the community.

Overall twice as many women consult for thyroid disorders and obesity but for diabetes the rates are the same in the two sexes.

Figure 40.2 shows the age distribution of consulting rates, with rates rising with age for diabetes and thyroid disorders but a peak at 25 for obesity.

Sickness–invalidity

2% of claims for certified sickness–invalidity benefits are for this group.

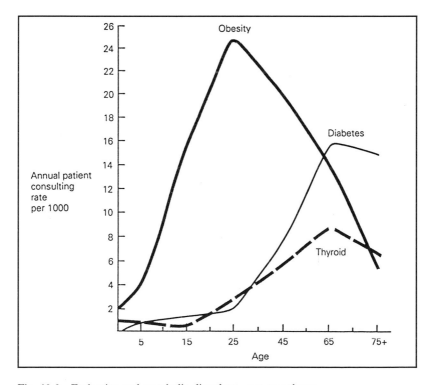

Fig. 40.2—Endocrine and metabolic disorders – age prevalence

Hospital data

> 2% of all admissions are for endocrine disorders – 2 per 10 000 for thyroid disorders and 10 per 10 000 for diabetes and its complications.
>
> Assuming that a collaborative district diabetic service is desirable, this means some 3000 diabetics per district general hospital.

Mortality

> Endocrine disorders are certified as causes of death in 8000 per year out of 600 000 in the UK (1.3%). Most (6000) are diabetics.

Clinical implications

As noted, planned care is required for these conditions.

- *Diabetes* (see Chapter 41): good shared care between general practice and the district specialist unit is the ideal.
- *Thyroid disorders* (see Chapter 42) also require long-term planned care. Early diagnosis demands keen clinical acumen by GPs and it is by no means easy to pick out the likely specific cause from amidst the multitude of similar non-specific symptoms. Once diagnosed, both *hyperthyroid* (best managed initially in collaboration with a specialist) and *hypothyroid* patients (can be managed by GPs alone) demand long-term supervision with annual checks on thyroid formation and attention to any medication dosage.
- *Obesity* is presumed to be the result of overindulgence and is linked with smoking and alcoholism as a personal social and behavioural problem. However, the precise causes and pathophysiology are uncertain. Whilst diagnosis is obvious, successful long-term weight reduction is difficult to attain and maintain.

CHAPTER **41**

DIABETES

What is it?

- One of the most important of chronic disorders requiring long-term supervision and support for the remainder of a person's life.
- A disorder of carbohydrate metabolism associated with relative or absolute deficiency of insulin.
- Over 1% of the population are diabetic and another 0.5%–1% are potential or undiagnosed diabetics.
- Diabetes affects more than the diabetic:
  family
  occupation and employers
  GP primary care team
  hospital – any department
  community services
  research workers
  drug companies

The *challenges* are to provide long-term care, control the elevated blood sugar, maintain normal function and good health and prevent complications.

Types

I   *Insulin dependent* (IDDM) is more severe; little or no endogenous secretion of insulin and therefore requiring insulin replacement; more prevalent in young persons with peaks at ages 5 and 12–18 (equal sex distribution).

II *Non-insulin dependent* (NIDDM) – mature onset and associated with obesity (females more than males); insulin still being produced naturally.

Diabetes is a genetically-predisposed condition.

It is due to damage to the beta-cells of the pancreas in the Islets of Langerhans, probably as a result of a combination of infection and toxic environmental factors, in a predisposed individual. Possible infections include Coxsackie B and rubella. The damaged beta-cells release protein which then produces auto-antibodies to the cells, and when > 80% of the beta-cells in the Islets of Langerhans are destroyed clinical diabetes develops.

In NIDDM there is deposition of amyloid material in the Islets of Langerhans.

Impaired glucose tolerance

There is another category of *impaired glucose tolerance* which occurs in patients who do not have clinical diabetes but do have the following results after a standard 75 g glucose tolerance test:

fasting blood sugar < 140 mg/dl;
30, 60 or 90 minute blood sugar > 200 mg;
2 h blood sugar 140–200 mg.

Although these patients are not overt diabetics when they are detected, 2–4% annually do develop unequivocal diabetes.

Aetiology of IDDM

The main factors are:

- genetic
- immunological
- hormonal
- environmental

Genetic

Increased frequency of HLA DR3 and HLA DR4.
Increased incidence of diabetes in siblings.

Immunological

Islet cell antibodies present in the early stages of the disease.

Immune-suppression with cyclosporin A soon after the onset of the diabetes can produce lasting remission of IDDM.

Environmental

Viral infection is the commonest 'trigger' in genetically-predisposed individuals.

Breast-feeding can offer some protection against the development of diabetes.

Aetiology of NIDDM

- *Genetic factors* – probably even more important than in IDDM. More twins are both affected by this diabetes than occurs in IDDM.
- *Insulin resistance.*
- *Abnormal beta-cell function* – evidence of abnormal beta-cell function is present in many of these patients, though insulin secretion is not significantly impaired.
- *Environmental factors*:
  obesity
  physical inactivity
  diet – a possible factor is inadequate fibre intake.

Who gets it and when?

As noted, national (UK) prevalence is over 1% (600 000) with another 0.5% (300 000) as potential or undiagnosed diabetics.

Age at first diagnosis

The incidence increases with age (Figure 41.1 and Table 41.1) but it occurs at all ages.

TABLE 41.1   Diabetes: age at first diagnosis (% of cases)

Age	0–9	10–19	20–29	30–39	40–49	50–59	60–69	70+
%	1.3	3.3	10	13	13	13	26	20

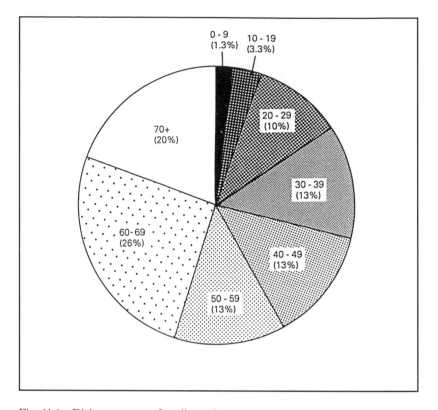

Fig. 41.1—Diabetes – age at first diagnosis

The *age prevalence* (Table 41.2 and Figure 41.2) shows an *increase* with age.

TABLE 41.2   Diabetes: age prevalence

Age	0–9	10–19	20–29	30–39	40–49	50–59	60–69	70+
per 1000	1	3	4	5	10	12	25	35

The *patient consulting rates* in practice (Table 41.3) show numbers that occur and need to be cared for.

A *district general hospital* can expect to be responsible for 2500 diabetics in collaboration with GPs.

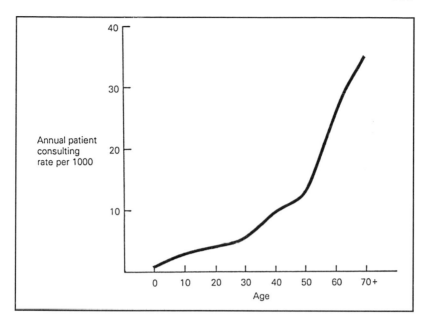

Fig. 41.2—Diabetes – age prevalence

TABLE 41.3   Diabetics in practices of 2000 and 10 000

	per 2000	per 10 000
Annual incidence (new cases)	2–3	10–15
Annual prevalence (persons consulting)	20–30	100–150
'Potential diabetics'	25	125
Total in practice	45–55	225–275

How does it present?

IDDM presentation

Severe acute diabetes:

- dehydration
- nausea and vomiting
- abdominal pain
- circulatory collapse
- stupor → coma.

Subacute diabetes:

- polyuria and polydipsia
- loss of weight
- fatigue and weakness
- pruritus
- paraesthesiae
- visual disturbances.

NIDDM presentation

- Many are asymptomatic and picked up on routine urine testing.
- Symptoms are often mild and gradual – thirst, polyuria and loss of weight developing over several months.
- Other symptoms:
  susceptibility to staphylococcal skin infections
  candida vaginitis
  balanitis.
- There is an increased mortality from atherosclerotic complications with a reduction of life expectancy of 5 to 10 years in a middle-aged patient.

Distinguishing features of IDDM compared with NIDDM

- Earlier age of onset.
- Prone to ketonuria.
- Normal or low body weight.
- Lower family incidence.
- IDDM present in close relatives.
- Islet cell antibodies present.
- HLA antigens B8, B15, DR3, DR4.

Diagnostic tests for diabetes

- Fasting venous plasma glucose > 7.8 mmol/l.
- Non-fasting venous plasma glucose > 11.1 mmol/l.
- If still doubtful do simple oral glucose tolerance test – 2 h after 75 g of glucose
  < 7.8 is normal
  > 11.1 is diabetes
  in between is impaired glucose tolerance.

Management of diabetes

Management is long-term and requires planning with protocols and guidelines and is best through shared care between general practice (primary care) and local specialist units.

Management of IDDM

Since survival in diabetes depends primarily on the presence or absence of vascular complications, the main aim of treatment is to prevent the development of both macrovascular and micro-vascular complications of diabetes. This prevention is determined by the quality of the blood sugar control.

In practical terms, therefore, the objectives of treatment are:

- to relieve symptoms – fatigue, thirst, polyuria and loss of weight;
- to prevent or delay complications – may be possible with retinopathy, neuropathy and nephropathy;
- to prolong life.

The essential components of effective treatment are:

- education
- diet
- insulin.

Education is a vital part of successful treatment in both IDDM and NIDDM.

The patient and close relatives must be made fully aware of the nature and possible course of the diabetes, the goals of treatment, the main complications and their possible prevention.

He should be instructed in treatment with diet, tablets or insulin, and how to cope with the acute complications like hypoglycaemia and keto-acidosis.

He should learn to monitor his own blood sugar with BM stix and keep a record.

Adequate foot care is essential to prevent long-term complications.

Most important, he should be made fully aware of when and where to seek expert medical advice.

Diet: Food intake is matched to insulin requirements.

5–6 meals/day may be necessary in some patients.

Total fat is reduced to 30% of total calories and cholesterol intake to < 300 g/day.

High fibre slows glucose absorption and is beneficial in reducing large swings of blood sugar.

Total calorie intake depends on physical activity.

Insulin – the main aim of insulin treatment is to maintain normoglycaemia:

- blood sugar 3.8–8.8 mmol/l before meals;
- glycosylated haemoglobin level within normal range.

Intermediate-acting insulins once or twice/day are not usually adequate to maintain normoglycaemia. Multiple injections of insulin mixtures combined with self-monitoring of blood sugar is probably the best regime to produce normoglycaemia, but may be impracticable in many patients especially the elderly, or shift workers.

A practical regime might be a combination of isophane and soluble insulins 2 or 3 times a day. The insulin should be given about 30 to 45 minutes before a meal.

Insulin pumps delivering a continuous supply of parenteral insulin offer advantages in blood sugar control, but are expensive and prone to breakdown. Also, they do not incorporate blood sugar sensing mechanisms, so hypoglycaemia or keto-acidosis can easily occur.

Complications of insulin therapy

- *Hypoglycaemia:*
  excessive dose of insulin
  delay in having meal
  excessive exercise.
- Keto-acidosis:
  infection is commonest cause
  myocardial infarction or stroke
  inadequate dose of insulin.
- Fat atrophy:
  at site of injection
  due to a local immune reaction
  treat by using highly refined insulin.
- Local allergic reaction at injection site – treat by changing to human insulin.
- Insulin resistance due to:
  abnormal metabolic response
  circulating IgG antibodies.
  may respond to immune suppression or to a change of insulin.

Unstable IDDM

- Occurs in 1% of diabetics.

- Rapid changes from hypoglycaemia to hyperglycaemia with keto-acidosis.
- Causes behavioural problems.
- Causes insulin problems:
  wrong dose
  variable absorption
  increased breakdown
  insulin antibodies.
- Causes autonomic neuropathy with resultant fall in sensory detection of symptoms of hypoglycaemia.

Management of NIDDM

General

- Check for and treat commonly associated conditions:
  obesity
  hypertension
  hyperlipidaemia
  vascular disease, e.g. claudication.
- Stop smoking.
- Foot hygiene and foot care.
- Check for and treat retinopathy.
- Check for renal disease including micro-albuminuria.
- Reduce or stop any diabetogenic drugs, e.g. steroids or thiazides.

Specific treatment

Diet – try dieting first in any obese patients.

Drugs – two groups of drugs are commonly used – biguandides and sulphonylureas. The biguanide, metformin, is used initially in obese patients, and a sulphonylurea in non-obese patients.

Metformin:

- Acts by decreasing hepatic glucogenesis (the production of glucose from glycogen), and it also increases tissue sensitivity to insulin. Metformin does not increase insulin secretion.
- Patients tend to lose weight.
- Hypoglycaemia is very rare.
- Does not cause lactic acidosis – unlike phenformin.
- Gastro-intestinal side-effects in up to 50% – nausea, dyspepsia and diarrhoea – usually transient only.

Sulphonylureas:

- Act by increasing insulin secretion.
- May increase patient's weight.

- First-line treatment in non-obese patients who are poorly controlled by diet and exercise.
- May lead to hypoglycaemia 4 or more hours after food – especially with glibenclamide in elderly patients.
- Minor gastro-intestinal side-effects.
- Particular side-effects with chlorpropamide:
  prolonged hypoglycaemia
  flushing
  palpitations especially with alcohol
  syndrome of inappropriate secretion of anti-diuretic hormone.

Indications for insulin in NIDDM

- Poor blood sugar control with diet and oral drugs.
- Persistently elevated Hb-A (glycosylated haemoglobin) which is a good indicator of unsatisfactory diabetic control and a persistently raised blood sugar in the previous 6 weeks.
- Unacceptable lethargy on existing treatment.
- Continued weight loss.
- Persistent ketonuria.

Although it is current practice to give insulin in the circumstances above, it is worth noting that many of these 'resistant' IDDM patients have more than adequate insulin levels in their blood: furthermore, giving more insulin may enhance the development of atherosclerosis.

Follow-up in patients with NIDDM

Regular follow-up is desirable in these patients because of the likely development of atherosclerotic complications, and because of the possibility of loss of diabetic control with diet and drugs alone. This follow-up can be done ideally on the basis of shared care between the general practitioner and hospital specialist – the GP could see the patient every 3 or 4 months for routine follow-up, and a more detailed check (with appropriate investigations or specialist referrals if necessary) could be done annually at the hospital.

The particular points to check in these regular reviews include:

- weight and blood pressure
- blood sugar control
- urine examination for ketones and albumin (including micro-albuminuria)

- symptoms and signs of any complications especially vascular disease:
  eyes – acuity, retinopathy, cataracts
  feet – infection, nail care, pulses, evidence of neuropathy.

What happens?

Diabetics are managed by:

• diet alone	30%
• diet and drugs	40%
• insulin	30%

Diabetics have *excess mortality rates* – 3-fold compared with non-diabetics. Those on insulin have 5-fold excess.

Excess causes of death in diabetics are from:

- ischaemic heart disease;
- renal failure;
- infections.

However, mortality rates have been declining over the past 25 years.

Morbidity

Most diabetics develop some complications if the disorder exists for over 15–20 years but now many are preventable by early diagnosis and therapeutic intervention.

Complications therefore are related to:

- degree of control
- duration of disorder
- type of diabetes
- age of diabetic.

Eyes

Cataract – both specific and non-specific, is more prevalent in diabetics.

Retinopathy:

- overall in 10–15% diabetics
- in those with a history of diabetes for over 20 years – 65% have retinopathy

- 8% of diabetics are blind (commonest cause of blindness at age 30–64)
- with modern management (laser coagulation) in 70% deterioration should be preventable.

Kidneys

Earliest abnormality is *microalbuminuria* which can lead on to macroproteinuria and glomerulosclerosis and renal failure.
After 20 years of diabetes:

- 15% have proteinuria and ¾ of these will suffer terminal renal failure.

Feet

After 20 years:

- 8% have no foot pulses
- 3% experience intermittent claudication
- less than 1% develop gangrene.

Neuropathy

After 20 years most have some neuropathy:

- feet at risk in   25%
- male impotence in 50%
- severe symptoms in 5%

Control of diabetes

Overall (blood sugar below 8–11 mmol)

- good   40%
- fair   40%
- poor   20%

Pregnancy

A dilemma occurs with the 1 in 4 women who are found to have glycosuria on routine testing [with no past history of diabetes]. These should have a blood glucose check and, if it is raised, a GTT and probably advice on a low-fat low-carbohydrate diet.
In the great majority the abnormal GTT returns to normal after pregnancy but may recur in subsequent pregnancies.

Practical points

- Two types of diabetes are recognized:
  insulin dependent diabetes mellitus (IDDM) with no production of endogenous insulin, mostly young onset and requiring lifelong insulin replacement
  non-insulin dependent diabetes mellitus (NIDDM), mature onset with some secretion of insulin; treated by diet and drugs if necessary.
- A potential pre-diabetic state exists with impaired glucose tolerance tests.
- Prevalence is approximately 1.5% or 30 diabetics per practice of 2000, 2–3 new cases each year and perhaps up to 20 undiagnosed potential or pre-diabetics.
- IDDM can present as an *acute* emergency with severe dehydration, vomiting, abdominal pain, shock and coma, if untreated; or *subacute* with weight loss, polyuria, thirst, weakness and vaginal or penile thrush.
- NIDDM is often asymptomatic or with only vague symptoms of non-health.
- Aims of management must be to control metabolic disturbances, maintain health and prevent complications through education of the diabetic and family, diet, drugs or insulin.
- IDDM on insulin – target blood sugar 3.8–8.8 mmol.
- NIDDM – general measures are to reduce weight, control high blood pressure and high lipids and avoid smoking, drugs if diet is unsuccessful and some may need insulin.
- Long-term care requires planning and shared care between the general practice and local specialists with regular (at least twice a year) checks of blood sugar, blood pressure, urine for microalbuminuria, eyes for retinopathy and feet.
- In general practice 30% of diabetics are managed with diet, 40% with drugs and 30% with insulin.
- Mortality is higher than expected in diabetics from IHD, renal failure and infections.
- Some complications are almost inevitable after 15–20 years, Most prominent are failing vision (retinopathy or cataract) renal failure from glomerulo-sclerosis, peripheral vascular disease (feet) and neuropathy.
- Good control of hyperglycaemia is not easy – 40% are well controlled, in 40% control is fair and in 20% it is poor.

CHAPTER 42

THYROID DISORDERS

What are they?

- Disorders of the thyroid gland are important.
- They are not uncommon.
- They require acute clinical acumen for early diagnosis in order to achieve control.
- They require long-term supervision and management.

   There are three main disorders of relevance to GPs:

- Hyperthyroidism
  diffuse (Graves' disease)
  nodular (Plummer's disease)
  clinical effects due to excessive production of T4 and/or T3.
- *Hypothyroidism*
  post thyroiditis (autoimmune)
  post hyperthyroid therapies (iatrogenic)
  neonatal.
- *Cancer*
  Rare – 1 case in 15 years per GP, or 2–3 during a lifetime professional career.

Who gets it when?

- Females : males – 6 : 1.
- *Age at diagnosis*: at any age but most at 30–60 (Figure 42.1).
- *Neonatal*: with nationwide screening cases are found 1 per 3 500 births. This means (in theory) 1 case per 100 years per GP or 1 every 20 years per group.
- *Prevalence* (Table 42.1) shows that in a group practice the 50–55 patients with thyroid disease may require a regular mini-clinic for a once or twice a year check to ensure good control. In particular the post-hyperthyroxic may become hypothyroid.

TABLE 42.1 Thyroid diseases: incidence and prevalence

Thyroid disease	per 2000	per 10 000
Annual incidence (new cases)		
Hyperthyroid	1 every 2 years	5 every 2 years
Hypothyroid	1 every 2 years	5 every 2 years
Total	1 per year	5 per year
Persons consulting annually (prevalence)		
Hyperthyroid	5	25
Hypothyroid	6	30
Total	11	55
Thyroid cancer	1 every 15 years	1 every 3 years
Neonatal hypothyroid	1 every 100 years	1 every 20 years

How do they present?

Hyperthyroidism

Common causes:

- Graves' disease (exophthalmic goitre) – due to autoimmune antibodies which interact with the thyroid stimulating hormone receptors resulting in either inhibition or stimulation of these receptors; these antibodies are found in 85–90% of all patients with clinical Graves' disease.
- toxic multinodular goitre
- toxic adenoma
- post-partum thyrotoxicosis.

Symptoms:

- Heat intolerance

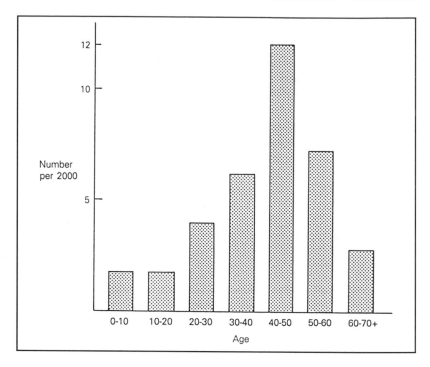

Fig. 42.1—Thyroid disorders – age at first diagnosis

- excessive sweating
- nervousness and tremors
- loss of weight with good appetite
- palpitations
- swelling of the neck
- staring eyes.

    Less common symptoms:

- diarrhoea
- oligomenorrhoea
- muscle weakness due to myopathy – more frequent in elderly patients
- psychosis.

Signs:

- fine tremor of the fingers
- hot, moist, 'silky' skin
- tachycardia

- goitre with systolic murmur over the gland (especially in Graves' disease)
- eye signs – exophthalmos, lid lag, etc.
- finger clubbing – rare
- pretibial myxoedema – rare.

Investigations:

A new sensitive immunometric assay of TSH can now distinguish between normal levels and the suppressed levels in thyrotoxicosis. This TSH assay is now all that is required in most patients with suspected hyperthyroidism.

Measurement of serum thyroxine levels are influenced by serum thyroglobulin levels, and misleading results can occur where the thyroglobulin level is altered, e.g. pregnancy, drugs (contraceptives, HRT, phenothiazines, phenytoin, etc.). It is therefore less reliable than the TSH level.

Thyroid scan with technetium-99 is useful in determining the nature of a goitre.

All thyroid nodules should have needle biopsy if diagnosis is not clear.

Treatment:

Block replacement therapy is the current effective method of treating thyrotoxicosis and avoids the need to continually monitor thyroid function and to titrate the dose of carbimazole as the patient progresses through the treatment:

- start with carbimazole 20 mg t.d.s.
- after 3–4 weeks when patient should be euthyroid reduce dose to 40 mg daily
- add thyroxine 100–150 micrograms daily to maintain euthyroidism
- discontinue treatment in 1 year.

Benefits of block replacement therapy:

- better compliance
- fewer visits to doctor
- better remission rate – however the rate of permanent remission with antithyroid drugs in Graves' disease is often only 50%. If there is a relapse, a further course of drugs is unlikely to be successful, so treatment should then be either subtotal thyroidectomy or radio-iodine if child-bearing is over.

Treatment of Graves' ophthalmopathy (malignant exophthalmos)

Severe progressive eye damage which can lead to blindness. The treatment available includes:

- high dose steroid therapy
- tarsorrhaphy
- orbital irradiation
- surgical decompression of the orbit.

Treatment of thyrotoxicosis in pregnancy

Propylthiouracil is a better antithyroid drug to use in pregnancy than carbimazole since it is less likely to cross the placental barrier and affect the foetus. This drug is also suitable for breast feeding.

Spontaneous remissions may occur in the last trimester.

An exacerbation of the thyrotoxicosis may also occur in the post-partum period.

Hypothyroidism

Symptoms:

- cold intolerance
- lack of energy
- weight gain
- constipation
- hoarse voice
- dry skin.

In elderly patients the presentation may be less clear:

- Cold intolerance and weight gain may be absent.
- Non-specific symptoms may be present:
  depression and confusion
  anorexia
  general exhaustion.

Signs:

- slow in thought and movement
- obesity
- coarse dry skin
- bradycardia
- slow relaxation of ankle jerks – useful sign
- signs of other autoimmune diseases, e.g. pernicious anaemia, rheumatoid arthritis, etc.

Investigations:

- measurement of TSH is the most reliable test – this is raised
- thyroid antibodies to thyroglobulin and the microsome can be measured since many patients with myxoedema, especially in the elderly, have Hashimoto's disease
- other tests:
  macrocytic anaemia
  abnormal liver function
  low serum Na levels.

Treatment of hypothyroidism

All patients should be treated even if the hypothyroidism is very mild.

The mainstay of treatment is thyroxine and it is rarely necessary to exceed a dose of 150 micrograms daily – treatment is lifelong.

If associated angina or heart failure is present the initial dose of thyroxine should be small, say 25 micrograms daily instead of the usual starting dose of 50 micrograms. Subsequent increase of dose should be determined by monitoring the TSH level, and increments made every 2 to 4 weeks.

When the patient is euthyroid, annual follow-up should be continued for life with annual checks of TSH levels which is the most reliable indicator of the thyroid state.

Subclinical hypothyroidism:

- Patient has no symptoms of hypothyroidism.
- TSH level is above normal.
- Thyroid antibody test may be positive.

These patients should be treated with thyroxine since most are inevitably going to become clinically hypothyroid sooner or later.

What happens?

Hyperthyroidism

- *Surgery* likely eventually for 4/5 of cases – correction of primary disorder but ½ – ⅓ will become *hypothyroid* over the years.
- *Drugs* – more than ½ relapse when drugs are stopped.
- *Radioactive iodine* – good control but ⅕ become *hypothyroid*.
- *No treatment* – a small proportion will settle naturally.

Hypothyroidism

Once definitive diagnosis has been made lifelong replacement therapy is necessary.

Note that autoimmune thyroid disorders may be associated with other autoimmune disorders, e.g. pernicious anaemia, Addison's disease.

Practical points

- In a practice of 2000 there are likely to be 6 persons with hypothyroidism (1 new case every 2 years) and 5 cases with hyperthyroidism (1 new case every 2 years). Thyroid cancer 1 case every 15 years and neonatal hypothyroidism 1 every 100 years!
- Best test for thyroid disorders is the TSH assay.
- Hyperthyroidism can be treated with block replacement by carbimazole. If control is achieved then treatment should be continued for at least one year and then stopped – but over one-half will recur and require thyroidectomy or radio-iodine therapy.
- Hypothyroidism may occur after treatment of hyperthyroidism.
- Hypothyroid patients require lifelong thyroxine replacement and twice yearly TSH checks to ensure good control.

SECTION X

MISCELLANEOUS

CHAPTER 43

SKIN DISORDERS – THE CLINICAL SPECTRUM

Since the skin is constantly exposed to the environment it is not surprising that skin disorders are a common group for consultation – 1 in 10 of all consultations.

However it must be realized that these consultations represent only a proportion of persons in the community with skin disorders, since most apply self-care.

Patient consulting rates

Over 18% of a practice population will consult for skin disorders annually (Table 43.1). This is one-quarter of all those who consult.

It is evident that *acute infections, warts* and *herpes*, are the largest group, followed by *eczema–dermatitis*. Note the relatively small numbers who consult for *acne*, this must represent barely one-tenth of the prevalence in the community. Note also that with minor surgery being promoted in general practice there can be many (25 per GP) sebaceous cysts, benign neoplasms and toe nail disorders, warts and abscesses to deal with.

TABLE 43.1   Annual consultation rates for skin disorders

	Persons consulting annually	
	per 2000	per 10 000
Acute infections	90	450
Herpes zoster	8	40
Herpes simplex	6	30
Eczema–dermatitis	100	500
Warts	30	150
Urticaria	16	80
Pruritus	14	70
Acne	20	100
Sebaceous cyst	10	50
Benign neoplasm	6	30
Malignant neoplasm	1	5
Psoriasis	10	50
Hair–nail disorders	15	75
Chronic ulcer	6	30
Pityriasis rosea	4	20
Napkin rash	10	50
Other	20	100

Who gets them and when?

There are differences in age and sex distributions for the various skin disorders (Table 43.2, Figure 43.1).

TABLE 43.2   Annual patient consulting rates per 1000 at various ages for selected skin disorders

Disease	Sex ratio	Age						
		0–4	5–14	15–24	25–44	45–64	65–74	75+
Acute infections	M = F	50	40	38	32	25	27	30
Warts	F > M	6	44	20	9	5	4	3
Herpes zoster	F > M	1	2	3	3	5	9	10
Herpes simplex		6	4	4	3	2	2	1
Eczema–dermatitis	M = F	110	42	52	30	30	33	35
Psoriasis	M = F	1	3	4	5	5	6	3
Acne	F > M	< 1	9	35	8	1	< 1	< 1
Urticaria	F > M	16	11	10	8	6	6	4
Nail – hair	M = F	5	8	11	5	5	6	5

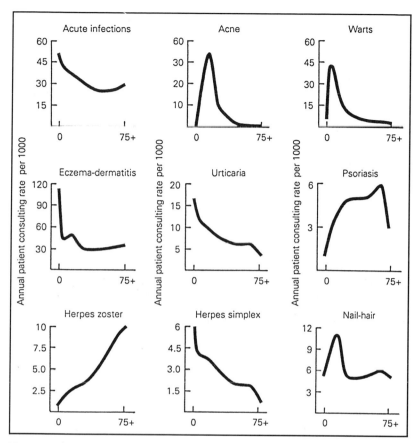

Fig. 43.1—Age prevalence of some specific skin disorders

Overall the highest consulting rates are in young children and teenagers, more in females than males.

- *Acute infections*: common in childhood but also in every age group.
- *Warts*: in schoolchildren and young adults.
- *Eczema–dermatitis*: in infancy, childhood and young adults but appreciable rates at all ages.
- *Psoriasis*: in adults of all age groups.
- *Acne*: in 15–25 age group.
- *Urticaria*: although all ages, most prevalent in children and young adults.
- *Herpes*: zoster rates rise with age; simplex most prevalent in childhood.

Skin disorders are responsible for very few hospital admissions, sickness absences or deaths.

CHAPTER 44

COMMON INFECTIONS – THE CLINICAL SPECTRUM

Whilst antibiotics and other modern lifesaving therapeutic measures have reduced deaths dramatically in developed countries, nevertheless, the prevalence of common infections in the community is very high – as has been noted in previous chapters.

Patient consulting rates

Taking all infections together, Table 44.1 shows that one-half of the population will consult in a year for some infection. It is the nature of general practice that the great majority will be 'non-specific' i.e. difficult to attribute to any specific pathogen.

As noted in Chapters 3, 20 and 43, upper respiratory infections are the largest group followed by gastro-intestinal and skin.

Sickness and invalidity

1 in 10 of all certified spells of sickness absence from work was for a common infection.

TABLE 44.1   Annual consultation rates for common infections

Disease (infections)	Annual patient consulting rates	
	per 2000	per 10 000
Non-specific		
Acute respiratory		
upper	444	2220
lower	128	640
Total	572	2860
Acute gastro-intestinal	136	680
Skin	120	600
Gynaecological	28	140
Urinary tract	60	300
Eye	72	360
Ear	92	460
Specific		
Whooping cough	6	30
Chicken pox	8	40
Measles	6	30
Rubella	6	30
Mumps	12	60
Glandular fever	4	20
Tuberculosis	1 every 5 years	1
Hepatitis	1	5
Meningitis	1 every 10 years	1 every 2 years

Hospital admissions

Only 3% of hospital admissions were for these conditions.

Causes of death

Whereas 35000 deaths in the UK each year are due to respiratory infections, including 1000 from tuberculosis, other infections, specific and non-specific, were responsible only for 2000 deaths.

CHAPTER 45

CANCER – THE CLINICAL SPECTRUM

Cancers cause one-quarter of all deaths annually (160 000 out of 650 000 in the UK), but they are not 'common'. Only 1 per cent of persons in a practice consult each year for cancer and they represent 10% of hospital admissions.

Cancers are important because they are life-threatening with only a 1 in 3 chance of a 5-year survival rate at present but probably this can be improved through early diagnosis and because it is estimated that 80% are preventable by avoidance of smoking and possible diet changes.

The GP has important roles in early diagnosis, prevention and terminal care when required.

Patient consulting rates

In a practice of 2000 there will occur 8 new cases of cancer each year (Table 45.1). In addition to these the GP will be consulted by another 12 in follow-up or terminal care.

418

TABLE 45.1   Cancers: annual numbers of new cases

Disease – cancer sites	New cases per year per 2000	per 10 000
All cancers	8	40
Lung	2 every 3 years	8
Breast	1	5
Skin	1	5
Gastro-intestinal		
Oesophagus	1 every 8 years ⎤	
Stomach	1 every 3 years ⎥	
Colon	1 every 2 years ⎥	5
Rectum	1 every 3 years ⎥	
Pancreas	1 every 5 years ⎦	
Urological		
Prostate	1 every 2 years ⎤	
Bladder	1 every 2 years ⎥	5
Kidney	1 every 10 years⎦	
Gynaecological		
Cervix	1 every 4 years ⎤	
Uterus	1 every 5 years ⎥	3
Ovary	1 every 4 years ⎦	
Leukaemia	1 every 5 years ⎤	
Brain	1 every 10 years⎥	
Myeloma	1 every 12 years⎥	less than 1
Testis	1 every 15 years⎥	
Hodgkin's lymphoma	1 every 20 years⎥	
Thyroid	1 every 20 years⎦	
Others	1	8

The distribution of the chief new cancers (Figure 45.1) is:

	% of total
Gastro-intestinal	24
Lung	17
Skin	12
Urinary	12
Breast	11
Gynaecological	6
Others	18

Sickness–invalidity

Cancers account for only 1.5% of claims.

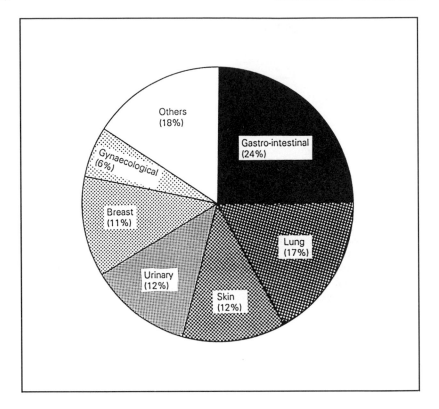

Fig. 45.1—Types of cancer

Hospital data

It is likely that a district general hospital servicing a 250 000 population can expect around 1000 new cancer referrals plus another 2000 follow-up cases.

Annual admissions for cancer are 10% of total.

Survival

Cancer Research Campaign data shows that 5-year survival rates for all cancers are almost 40% – (males 35% and females 46%)

The rates for some specific cancers are listed in Table 45.2.

TABLE 45.2   5-year survival rates for some cancers

Cancer site	% 5-year survival
Skin (including melanoma)	97
Uterus	72
Breast	64
Cervix	57
Ovary	27
Bladder	63
Prostate	43
Rectum	37
Colon	36
Stomach	10
Oesophagus	8
Leukaemia	30
Lung	8
Pancreas	4

[Cancer Research Campaign: Factsheets 1987–1992]

Table 45.3 shows the 5-year survival rates arranged in three groups with the 'best' more than one-half surviving more than 5 years; a 'moderate' group; and the 'worst' group with less than 10% chance of survival.

TABLE 45.3   % of persons with cancer surviving 5 years

50%+	49–10%	Less than 10%
Bladder	Bone	Gall bladder
Breast	Brain	Liver
Cervix	Colon	Lung
Eye	Kidney	Oesophagus
Hodgkin's lymphoma	Leukaemia	Pancreas
Larynx	Mouth	Stomach
Melanoma	Myeloma	
Other skin	Ovary	
Testis	Non-Hodgkin's lymphoma	
Thyroid	Pharynx	
Uterus	Prostate	
	Rectum	

[Cancer Research Campaign]

The Department of Health in *Health of the Nation 1991* suggests that:

- surgery alone cures 22% of cancers
- radiotherapy alone cures 12% of cancers
- surgery and radiotherapy cures 6% of cancers
- chemotherapy alone cures 2% of cancers
- chemotherapy plus other cures 3% of cancers

Deaths

There are 165 000 deaths from cancer net of 650 000 deaths a year in the UK. This is 5–6 per GP with 2000 patients (Table 45.4).

TABLE 45.4   Annual deaths from cancers in general practices

Sites	Annual deaths from cancer	
	per 2000	per 10 000
Lung	2	10
Breast	1 every 2 years	2–3
Prostate	1 every 3 years	1–2
Stomach	1 every 3 years	1–2
Colon	1 every 2 years	2–3
Rectum	1 every 5 years	1
Bladder	1 every 7 years	less than 1
Pancreas	1 every 5 years	1
Leukaemia	1 every 8 years	less than 1
Cervix	1 every 15 years	1 every 3 years
Ovary	1 every 7 years	less than 1
Uterus	1 every 20 years	1 every 4 years
Total	5–6	25–30

CHAPTER 46

ACCIDENTS – THE CLINICAL SPECTRUM

It is difficult to estimate the number of all accidents in the community. Certainly everyone sustains some 'accident' each year. Most are minor and self-treated but accidents are responsible for much work in hospital and general practice.

Hospitals deal with many more accidents than GPs, all major and many minor accidents. Thus 25% of the population now attend hospital accident–emergency (AE) departments annually. This means 500 patients in a practice of 2000 compared with the 240 others who see their GP. This suggests that perhaps one-third of the population seek treatment for accidents annually.

Table 46.1 shows the numbers and types of accidents seen in general practice annually.

Note that strains, sprains, bruises, contusions and lacerations account for most.

Sickness–invalidity

Only 5% of certified spells of sickness-absence are for accidents.

Hospital data

As noted, almost 1 in 4 of the population *attends AE departments* each year.

423

TABLE 46.1 Annual consultation rates for accidents

Accident – type	Annual consultation rates	
	per 2000	per 10 000
Sprains, strains	80	400
Soft tissue – bruises, etc.	50	250
Lacerations	40	200
Fractures	22	110
Head injuries	8	40
Burns	6	30
Insect bites	14	70
Other	40	200

Only 1–2% of the population are *admitted to hospital* for accidents in a year:

- fractures 43 per 10 000
- other accidents 100 per 10 000.

Causes of death

Almost 20000 deaths a year occur from accidents in the UK. This means 4–5 deaths per year in a practice of 10000 persons.

The causes are:

Road traffic accidents	5600
Home accidents	5000
Fires	1000
Suicide	4500
Homicide	400
Drug accidents	500
Other accidents and violence	3000
Total	20 000

CHAPTER 47

AGE – THE CLINICAL SPECTRUM

In other sections and chapters the emphasis has been on organ-systems and on common specific diseases. Here the accent will be on age-periods and on the common diseases that occur at the various times.

Patient consulting rates

Taking childhood, young adults, middle-age and old age as four periods the following are the *common diseases* (RCGP/OPCS, 1986) (Figure 47.1).

In *childhood* infections of all types are commonest but in particular respiratory, gastro-intestinal and skin infections and the specific fevers. Also figuring prominently will be conjunctivitis, acute otitis media and acute throat infections. Enuresis, constipation, eczema, warts, accidents and behaviour problems are also common.

In *young adults* the following are common – acute appendicitis, acne, infectious mononucleosis, warts, scabies, fungal infections, migraine, hay fever, cystitis, iron deficiency anaemias, gynaecological problems and family planning.

425

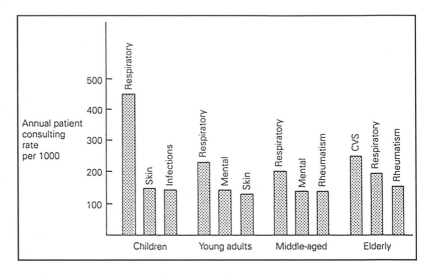

Fig. 47.1—Common diseases at various ages (top three)

In *middle-age* the common reasons for consultation are – anxiety-neurosis, depression, obesity, haemorrhoids, backache, anaemia, high blood pressure, coronary artery diseases and bronchitis.

In *old age* the most common diseases are – arthritis, bronchitis, heart failure, diabetes, gall bladder disorders, vertigo, constipation, insomnia, depression, high blood pressure, neoplasia, cataract, angina, cerebrovascular diseases, hernia and pernicious anaemia.

At all ages accidents, eczema, otitis externa, ear wax and asthma occur at equal rates.

Hospital admissions

Figure 47.2 shows the common reasons for hospitalization at the different ages. In *childhood* accidents, infections, respiratory diseases, gastro-intestinal disorders, ear diseases and endocrine, nutritional and metabolic disorders are the most likely reasons.

In *young adults* pregnancy, accidents, respiratory diseases and rheumatic, skin and gastro-intestinal disorders are the reasons.

In *middle-age* heart diseases, high blood pressure, cancer, gastro-intestinal disorders, rheumatism, respiratory diseases and accidents are the reasons.

In *old age* the chief reasons for hospitalization are – heart diseases, peripheral vascular disorders, cancers, bronchitis and pneumonia, accidents and gastro-intestinal diseases.

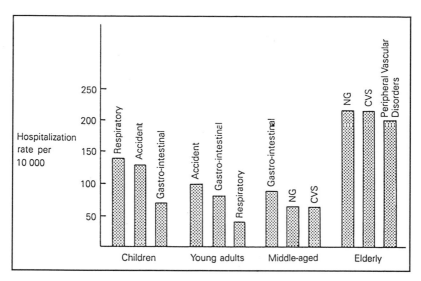

Fig. 47.2—Hospitalization – common causes (top three)

Deaths

Figure 47.3 shows the most likely causes of death at the various ages.

The chief cause of death in *children* is accidents followed by infections and diseases of the respiratory system and cancer. As persons grow *older* the killer diseases become heart diseases, strokes, cancer, chest diseases and, yet again, accidents.

Challenges for the future

The epidemiological facts and data presented in this book must serve a constructive purpose. They must be used to formulate policies for better care in the future.

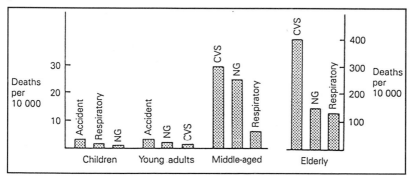

Fig. 47.3—Causes of death at various ages (top three)

In spite of the advances of medicine, morbidity has not declined. Common diseases still commonly occur and are likely to continue to do so in the future unless positive measures are taken to prevent them and to encourage efforts by the public to accept greater responsibilities for better health through better personal habits and behaviour.

At each age period there are certain actions that can be taken by the public and physicians to improve health and prevent disease.

Childhood

In developed countries *deaths* in children should be rare but in a practice population of 2500 persons in the United Kingdom there is one death every 2 years in an infant and one death every 4 years in children and young persons between 1 and 20 years of age. In infancy most deaths are due to prematurity and congenital defects. Prevention is related more to improving social conditions than to medical advances.

In the 1–20 age period, one-half of deaths are caused by accidents, a quarter by cancers and another quarter from respiratory and other infections. Certainly accidents are always preventable and deaths from infections could be.

There has been no reduction in *morbidity* from acute illnesses in childhood. The severity has declined but the prevalence is unaltered. Respiratory infections, other infections, skin disorders and accidents are the common causes of morbidity. Many are not preventable but some infections can be controlled by antibiotics and some can be prevented by widescale immunization. To achieve better health, a service of regular child care with an easily accessible and available personal service must be created in primary care.

In an average practice there will be some children who will suffer from *recurrent and chronic conditions* such as asthma (10 per 2500), epilepsy (3), urinary tract infections (3), diabetes (1), cystic fibrosis (1), coeliac disease (1), and enuresis (possibly up to 30 children).

Childhood should be the period when good health habits are inculcated and bad habits prevented. It is the period when good health education should discourage smoking (but over one-third of 16-year-old children in the UK smoke), discourage abuse of alcohol and over-eating and encourage regular exercise, weight control and dental hygiene.

Adult life

The primary physician, the family doctor, will be consulted by almost all of his adult patients at least once every 5 years. These regular consultations should be used for more than dealing with the presenting problems. They should serve to record certain basic clinical data (at least once every 5 years), to enquire on personal health, habits and behaviour. They should provide opportunities also to offer advice on personal measures that might be taken to improve health and to prevent disease.

The age period 20–45 is the time *before* the major diseases occur. It is the time before cardiovascular and cerebrovascular disorders occur, before cancer strikes and before degenerative changes in the jonts occur. It may be that preventive measures can be taken.

The *basic minimal clinical data set* should include records of height, weight, blood pressure and urine – perhaps with vision and hearing and checks of haemoglobin and blood fats – every 5 years.

However, there is no reliable evidence that 'medical check-ups' of themselves will prevent anything. They must be used with critical discrimination to influence personal patient behaviour and to correct correctable disorders if, and when, they are discovered.

The aged

Multiple pathology is the norm in the elderly. It must be accepted that physical and mental abnormalities will be detected in all persons over 65. The ageing mind and body become worn and liable to the common diseases of ageing, namely heart failure, effects of coronary artery occlusion, effects of narrowing of cerebral arteries and of other peripheral arteries in the legs, eyes, kidneys and gut, respiratory failure from 'chronic bronchitis and emphysema', rheumatism and arthritis, and cancers.

An optimistic medical philosophy is essential in good care of old persons. The emphasis must be on maintaining optimal function rather than on attempts to cure non-curable processes of ageing.

The old person must be cared for as a whole with as much attention paid to social conditions and to morale as to correction of correctable medical disorders.

The care of the aged is as much a part of good family medical care as is child care and arrangements must be made to provide easily available access for elderly patients to the physician and his team. A balance has to be struck towards appropriate care. Over-care of the elderly may be as bad as under-care. The elderly must be helped to live at terms with their inevitable disabilities. False hopes must not be raised but false pessimism and missed opportunities must also be avoided.

Death and dying

The mortality of life is 100%. We shall all die because we must, because we have been born. We all of us seek to live long and die well.

The life expectancy in developed countries is now well over the biblical three score and ten years. The improvements in life expectancy have been largely because of safer childbirth and safer childhood and better living and social conditions. The life expectancies of men and women who have reached middle-age have gone up little over the past quarter of a century.

In the United Kingdom only one-third of those who die do so at home. Twenty-five years ago it was one-half.

It is likely that about one-quarter of all deaths are quick, and unexpected, occurring in a matter of minutes or hours. In another one-quarter the final illness lasts less than a month. In one-half the process of dying is more prolonged and requires planning of care for the individual and family.

Death is a personal affair with the family involved. The principles of good care of the dying must be to treat the individual as a person in need of humane and human care and attention. Personal moral and religious views must be respected. Fears and anxieties must be allowed to surface and tackled honestly. Pains and discomfort must be relieved with all the many measures that are available. It is in the care of the dying that good nursing can render the greatest comfort. Powerful pain-relieving drugs must be used with courage and discrimination when indicated. All pains can be controlled with drugs. In the dying there must be no fear or anxieties in using potent addictive drugs. The dying have little time to become addicted.

The family of the dying must be supported before and after death. The period of bereavement is hard to bear and can be made more bearable by offers of support from the family physician, but the support must not be overwhelming. Each family will bear its grief and bereavement in its own ways.

Medical support can be helpful in explanation, in providing outlets in discussion, in providing guidance and advice on the future and in helping with material matters such as finance, sedation, certification, etc.

Ageing – future research

Free oxygen radicals and ageing

There is substantial evidence that ischaemic tissue, i.e. organs and tissues deprived of an adequate blood supply as a result of arterial disease, produces 'oxygen radicals', which can react with and damage cell membranes in their vicinity (lipid peroxidation), resulting in cell death. There is evidence available that cell damage by these toxic free oxygen radicals can contribute to the development of a number of the common diseases associated with ageing, e.g. ischaemic heart disease, cerebrovascular disease, degenerative and inflammatory joint disease, emphysema and Parkinson's disease.

There are a number of endogenous and exogenous free radical 'scavengers' which can inhibit the activity of these toxic radicals. Endogenous scavengers include the enzymes superoxide dismutase and catalase which prevent further ischaemic damage by the radicals. Exogenous substances which can 'scavenge' free radicals include vitamin C and vitamin E, beta-carotene (present in red fruits and vegetables) and a new group of steroid compounds called lazaroids. Current research is now under way to see whether any of these free radical scavengers or anti-oxidant agents can prevent the cell damage which is the result of the ishaemia occurring inevitably in the ageing process. This work does not constitute the 'elixir of eternal youth', a concept much sought after by the philosophers of old, since all the body cells are genetically programmed for a specific life span, and it is highly unlikely that this can ever be altered, but this research may have exciting possibilities for retarding or preventing some of the crippling diseases accompanying old age.

INDEX

432